Responsiveness in Music Therapy Improvisation

Karette Stensæth

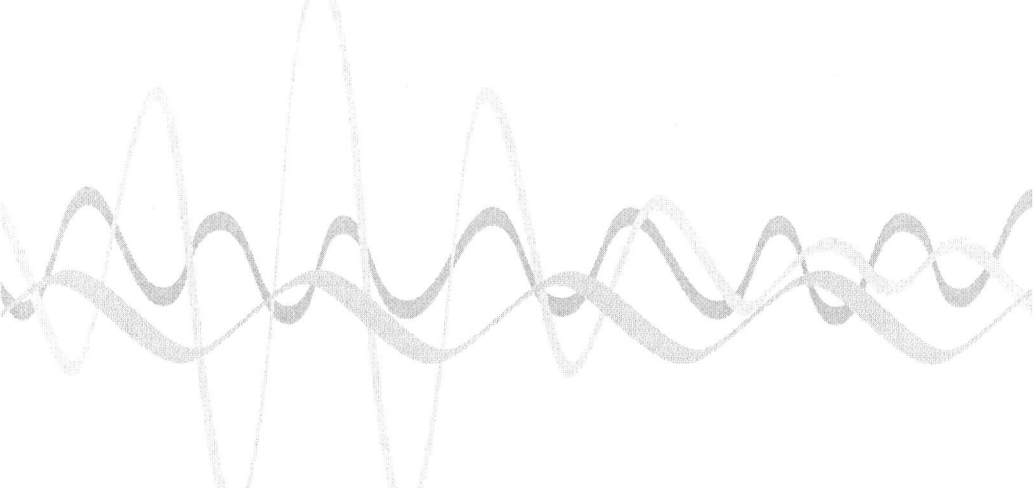

A Perspective Inspired by Mikhail Bakhtin

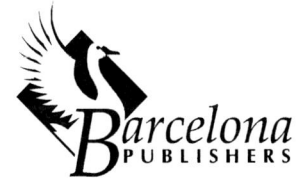

Responsiveness in Music Therapy Improvisation:
A Perspective Inspired by Mikhail Bakhtin

© 2017 Barcelona Publishers

All rights reserved. No part of this book may be reproduced,
stored, distributed, or sold in any form whatsoever.
For permissions, contact
Barcelona Publishers.

Print ISBN: 9781945411236
E-ISBN: 9781945411243

Barcelona Publishers
10231 Plano Road
Dallas TX 75238
www.barcelonapublishers.com
SAN 298-6299

Cover design: © 2017 Frank McShane

Copy-Editor: Jack Burnett

This book is a celebration of laughter, struggle, uncertainty, and openness in music therapy.

ACKNOWLEDGMENTS

I owe many people gratitude. I am grateful to Lars Ole Bonde, who, as my mentor, first encouraged me to contact Barcelona Publishers with the book proposal. I thank Kenneth Bruscia for his quick and inspiring response on the idea! I am grateful for many inspiring dialogues with the esteemed group of researchers at CREMAH, the Centre for Research in Music and Health at The Academy of Music in Oslo. In addition to Lars Ole, these are Gro Trondalen and Even Ruud. I am also grateful for the collaboration with my colleagues in The International Consortium of Eight Universities. I owe gratitude to the academy, to my colleagues, and especially those in the music therapy program. They are Tone S. Kvamme, Rita Strand Frisk, Tom Næss, Bente Almås, Ruth Eckhoff, and Hans Petter Solli. I also want to thank my students and my friends at the academy. I am honored to be around so many warm, hardworking, skilled, and dedicated people there. A very special thank you to Jakob, the client in the narrative used for this book. I will never forget our music therapy improvisations! I owe my big family a gratitude. Heartfelt thanks go to my precious children, Regine, Fridtjof, and Mathea, and to their continuous re-creation of wonderful carnivalesque moments in my life. Thanks to Bjørn Kruse for his very helpful proofreading of the language in the final stages. I am of course grateful to the legacy of Mikhail Bakhtin. His ideas have changed my thinking about so many things. Indirectly, they have changed my life, too. My husband and I "found" each other as we discussed Bakhtin's ideas on music, Being, and Dialogue. Bjørn: Thanks for everything and for being so beautifully answerable with your whole life. This book is for you and the people we love.

TABLE OF CONTENTS

Acknowledgments iv
Table of Contents v
List of Figures xii
Prelude xiii
Introduction 3
    The Book's Scope 4
        An Indigenous Ideal? 4
        An Insider Perspective 5
    Personal and Professional Context 5
        Clinical Background 6
        My Preunderstanding 7
        A Personal (Musical) Narrative 8
        The Structure of the Book 11

Chapter 1: (Re)Defining Core Concepts 13
    Responsiveness 13
    Music Therapy 14
        Dialogues on Music Therapy 15
        The Difficult Words 16
    Health 17
    Music Therapy Improvisation 17
        Music Therapy Improvisation in the Nordoff-Robbins Tradition 18
    Music Therapist 22
        A Supportive Teacher, a Helper, and a Creative Musician 22
        A Companion and an Accompanist 23
        A "Mother?" 23
        A Participating Observer and a Personal Motivator 24
        The Music Therapist's Relationship to the Music 24
        The Role of Action in the Music Therapist's Approach 24
        Summing up the Definition of "Music Therapist" 25
    Client 26
        Client as a Field of Beauty 26
        Client as Engager 27
        Client as Collaborator 27
    Meaning 27

    Hallgjerd Aksnes and Even Ruud on Meaning 28
    Musical Meaning 28
    Meaning as Action 29
    Dialogical Meaning-Making 29
Time 29
    David Aldridge's Perspective on *Chronos* and *Kairos* 30
    Musical Time 30
    Time as Communicative Musicality 31
    "Participatory Discrepancies" 31
    A Place with Groove 32
    Even Ruud Transposing Victor Turner's "Communitas" 32
    "We" in Alfred Schütz's manner 33
Aesthetics 33
    Art as Symbols in Suzanne Langer's View 34
    Bjørn Kruse on Dramaturgy and Schiller's Play 35
Ethics in Donald Schön's Perspective 36
    Ethical Artistry 37
    Closeness ethics and/or Situational Ethics 37
Theory 37

CHAPTER 2: ACTION 39
Action and Socialization 39
    George Herbert Mead's Social Act 40
    Ivar Frønes on Socialization 40
    Daniel Stern on the Emergent Self 40
"To Increase Possibilities for Action" 41
Dag Østerberg on the Phenomenon of Action 42
    Action as a Dialectical Phenomenon 43
    The Anonymous Action 44
    The Unfolding Spontaneous Action 44
    Actions as a Means for an Intention 45
    A Practical View on Action 45
The Relationship between Action and Intention in Music Therapy Improvisation .. 46
Playful Action 47
    Aleksei Leontjev on Play 48
    Mihaly Csikszentmihalyi on Action Possibilities and Challenges 48
A Short Summing up on Action 48

CHAPTER 3: INTRODUCING THE MUSIC THERAPY NARRATIVE 49
    The Observations 49
        Differences between My Observation and the Other Observations 50
        The Logs 51
        The Image of Michelangelo's *Creation of Adam* 51
        Challenges Connected to My Merging of the Observations into One Narrative 52
        How to Read the Narrative 53
        The Structure of the Narrative 53

CHAPTER 4: THE NARRATIVE OF JAKOB AND KARLA 55
    The Guitar Excerpt 55
    The Djembe Excerpt 60
    Both Excerpts 66

CHAPTER 5: SUMMING UP THE NARRATIVE 69

CHAPTER 6: INTRODUCING MIKHAIL BAKHTIN AND HIS CONTEXT 73
    About Bakhtin 73
        The Basis of Dialogue 73
        Reading Bakhtin 74
        Who and What Inspired Bakhtin? 75
        The Bakhtin Circles 75
        Lived Experiences? 76

CHAPTER 7: CONCERNING MY TRANSPOSING OF INSIGHTS OF BAKHTIN'S IDEAS 77
    My Perspective 77
        Bringing Bakhtin's Ideas into Dialogue with Other Traditions 77
        Communicative Being and Communicative Repairing 78
        United in a Pragmatically Oriented Science Philosophy 79

CHAPTER 8: MIKHAIL BAKHTIN'S TERMINOLOGY 81
    Answerability 81
        Answerability and Addressivity 82
        Answerability as Active Engagement 83
    Dialogue 83
        Dialogue Inspiration 83
        Influences from Buber's Dialogue 84
        Dialogue as Existence 84
    Other Related Concepts 85
        Bakhtin's Action 85

Relation 85
The Other 86
Bakhtin's Architectonic Model of the Human Psyche 87
The Utterance 87
Heteroglossia 88
Voices and Polyphony 89
Ventriloquism 90
Authorship 91
Carnival 91
Carnival's Ability to Regenerate and Revitalize Life 92
Laughter 92
A Short Summing Up of Bakhtin's Ideas 94

Chapter 9: Bakhtin's Ideas on Dialogue, Transposed to Responsiveness in Music Therapy Improvisation 97

Responsiveness in Music Therapy Improvisation 98
Two Levels of Responsiveness 99
Dialogical Responsiveness 99
Responsiveness as Dialogue 99
Responsiveness as a Multivoiced Activity 100
Responsiveness as Exploration 100
Jakob and Karla Exploring Responsiveness 100
Strangeness in the Responses—and Client and Therapist as Strangers 101
Strangeness as Tension 102
Unfinalized Responses and Unfinalizable Individuals 102
Comparisons with Other Philosophers 103
Mikhail Bakhtin versus Martin Buber and Emmanuel Levinas 103
Bakhtin and Buber 104
Bakhtin and Levinas 104
The Differences Between Bakhtin, Levinas, and Buber 105

Chapter 10: Bakhtin's Ideas on Answerability, Transposed to Responsiveness in Music Therapy Improvisation 107

Responsiveness and Answerability 108
Panagiotis Kanellopoulos on the "Oughtness" to Act 108
The "Ought" in Music Therapy Improvisation 110
The Musical-Relational "Ought" Exemplified with Jakob and Karla 110
Music as the Spark of a Musical-Relational Answerability 111
The Music Therapist's Responsibility 112
Answerability in a Professional Sense 113
Answerability in a Personal Sense 113

Stepping Outside and Reflect-in-Action 114
Searching for (Dialogical) Meaning 115
Helping the Client Becoming Response-able 116

CHAPTER 11: "WE:" A COMMUNITY OF MUSIC THERAPY IMPROVISATION 117
A Community of Music Therapy Improvisation 117
    A Community of Improvisation for Jakob and Karla 117
    Defining a Dialogical Agency in Each Other 118
    Monological Aspects 119
    Dialogue and Monologue as Complementary Aspects 119
    Vulnerable Relations and Face-to-Face Positioning 120
    Ethical Aspects in Vulnerable Relationships 120
    Responsiveness as a Human Capacity 121
    Being a "Close Other" 121
    To Doubt One's Own Voice 121
    Ulla Holck on Expectation 122
    An Ethical and Loving Responsiveness 122
    An Aesthetical Awareness in the I–You Relation 123
    Taking the Position of a Participant, not a Spectator 124
    Music as an Aesthetical Agent 124

**Chapter 12: BAKHTIN'S IDEAS ON CARNIVAL, TRANSPOSED
TO RESPONSIVENESS IN MUSIC THERAPY IMPROVISATION** 127
Carnival and Improvisation 127
    The Need for Carnival for Jakob and Karla 127
    Carnival as Democracy 128
    Carnival Characteristics 128
Kjetil Steinsholt's Carnival: Carnival as Play 129
    A World Upside Down 129
    In the Center of Here-and-Now 130
Summarizing the Main Aspects of "My" Carnival 130
Is the Music Therapist a Jester? 133

CHAPTER 13: MERGING PERSPECTIVES ON CARNIVAL, PLAYFULNESS, AND ACTION 135
Conditions for Responsiveness 135
    A Playlike Condition 135
    Carolyn Kenny on Play Conditions 136
    The Presence of Several Levels of Consciousness 136
Materializing Time Aspects in the Improvisation Between Jakob and Karla 137
    Delayed Synchronicity or/and Participatory Discrepancies 138
    Having a "Real" Discussion on the Djembe? 139

Action Versus Interaction 140
    Struggling with Actions and Each Other 140
    No First Initiative 141
Maintaining a Dialogical Mind-set in the Carnival 141
    The Dialogical Mind-set, seen from the Practical Level 142
    Jakob Making Question Mark with his Arms 142
    Upholding the Dialogical Mind-set 143
    Imagining the Other 143
    Karla Exploring Ventriloquism 145
Summing Up 146

Chapter 14: "Musical Answerability:" A Theory on Responsiveness in Music Therapy Improvisation Inspired by Bakhtin 149

Introducing My Theory 149
    Musical Answerability as a Dialogical Theory 150
    Musical Answerability as a Theory of Ethics 151
    Musical Answerability as a Theory of Aesthetics 152
Placing Musical Answerability within Three Perspectives 153
    Musical Answerability, an Existential Perspective 153
    Musical Answerability, a Social Perspective 153
    Musical Answerability, a Practical-Relational Perspective 154
    A Practical-Relational Understanding with a Body-Based Perspective 155
    A Practical-Relational Perspective with a Personal Imprint 155
    A Practical-Relational Perspective and its Use of Musical Parameters 156
Summarizing the Main Characteristics of the Theory 156

CHAPTER 15: DISCUSSING THEORY ASPECTS 161
    Musical Answerability as an Interlevel Theory 162
    Is the Theory Music-Centered? 163
    Returning to the Question of Authorship 164
        Authorial Comprehension 165

CHAPTER 16: A RETURN TO THE QUESTION, WHAT IS MUSIC THERAPY? 167
    Framing the Question 167
    Responsiveness and Musically Answerable Acts 169

POSTLUDE 171
NO LAST WORDS 174
REFERENCES 175
ATTACHMENTS 184
    The Guitar Excerpt 184
    The Guitar Excerpt, part 2 185
    The Djembe Excerpt 186
    The Djembe Excerpt, part 2 187
    The Djembe Excerpt, part 3 188
ENDNOTES 189

LIST OF FIGURES

Figure 1. The three work phases in the Nordoff-Robbins–oriented approach. 40
Figure 2. The action–intention axis. 71
Figure 3. Rhythmical development in the therapist's guitar-playing. 81
Figure 4. Swinging rhythm in the guitar-playing. 82
Figure 5. Varying the guitar rhythm. 82
Figure 6. Playing faster 85
Figure 7. Exchange of rhythm. 87
Figure 8. Longer interaction phrase. 88
Figure 9. Powerful strength and greater complexity. 89
Figure 10. Karla accompanies Jakob 89
Figure 11. "Materializing" time aspects. 173
Figure 12. Imagining the Other in The Guitar Excerpt. 180

PRELUDE

When a client who is a mystery to me enters the room and my task as his music therapist is to approach him musically and try to make something meaningful out of the situation, I immediately start acting and reflecting in certain ways. The uncertainty and struggle to find connections with him affect me as soon as I see his face. I try to grasp the feeling of him, his actions and playing, thus regarding his expressions as a source for my own responses. Many questions pop into my head: What do I feel when I see him? Should I act out my feelings or not? What does he feel? What could I expect from him? What does he expect from me? How should I start the music—and continue it? Softly? With fermatas, to open up? Or with rhythmical playing, to invite him into a groove? How does he respond to my playing? Does he like it—or dislike it? Does he want to join in? How could I welcome him into my music, my world? Does he invite me into his?

Perhaps a more overriding question might permeate my self-questioning when I start reflecting upon what happened. This question engages the philosophical Whys: Why did I do what I just did? Why did he do what he just did? Was it important in any way? Why? For whom was it important? And so forth.

As a music therapist, I have always felt that I explore existential topics together with my clients in music therapy improvisation: It is not just the music that we explore. It is not just each other whom we explore either. It is more than that: It is life itself and the meaning of life.

I have also felt that the improvisational approach in music therapy represents a unique and exciting—almost magnetic—way of exploring life and being in the here-and-now. Therefore, as a researcher in the field, I have asked myself: How can I understand my ideas and deep fascination with these aspects of music therapy improvisation? Is there any theory and/or philosophy that can "explain" my reflections?

I found some answers when I came across Mikhail Bakhtin's work. His ideas on dialogue, responsiveness, action, aesthetic, and ethics have inspired me enormously. As I have been working with this book, I have also come to realize how Bakhtin's worldview is linked to my own life and my lived experiences. I have therefore allowed myself to be personal in some parts of the book.

Now, reading Bakhtin and understanding his ideas is not easy. After my presentation of Bakhtinian perspectives in music therapy in the Bakhtin 2014 conference in Stockholm, I asked Bakhtin scholar Craig Brandist his opinions of my internalization of Bakhtin's ideas.[1] He said: "Wonderful and very interesting. Just be clear as to when your ideas take over Bakhtin's ideas." Brandist's advice helped me sort out some of my thoughts. I also talked to Eugene Matusov, another Bakhtin scholar, at the same conference.[2] He too applauded my work and invited me to become a member of the Dialogic Pedagogy Facebook page, which introduced me to many novel readings of Bakhtin. Both of them, without knowing it, inspired me greatly to continue my exploration of Bakhtin in my work.

The present book involves creative theory building on music therapy improvisation that does not necessarily apply to clinical practice. My wish, although without immediate obvious implications for what to do, is that my ideas will contribute to explicate new insight about music therapy improvisation and thereby indirectly influence music therapy practice.

In that it deals with the mix of Bakhtin, music, improvisation, human interaction, and quality of life, the book should be of interest to many people, areas, and professions. The topic should be relevant for music therapy, art, sociology, musicology, (music) education, (music) psychology, (music) philosophy, and so on. I hope that Bakhtin scholars have interest in it. Music therapists who love the mix of improvisation and philosophy should find it especially interesting: I hope that the book inspires you to love what you do even more.

Karette Stensæth
Oslo, Norway
June 15, 2017

Responsiveness in Music Therapy Improvisation

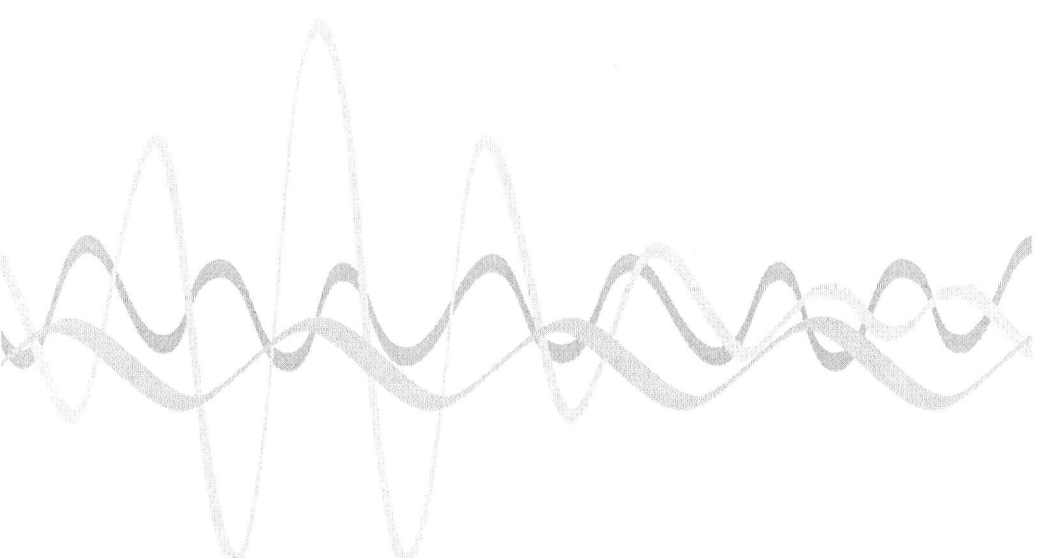

INTRODUCTION

Much of the material in the book is collected from my PhD work involving Bakhtin (Stensæth, 2008), but because I have continued to elaborate upon his ideas after that, the present book includes several new aspects. Its purpose is to outline novel perspectives on responsiveness in music therapy improvisation that might provide a fresh conceptual framework for the broad value of active and creative music-making in therapy. The last chapters present a theory on responsiveness in music therapy improvisation, which I have called Musical Answerability.

Because it deals with human processes such as interpretation and understanding, the book places itself within the field of hermeneutics. It also resonates with a humanistic tradition, which pervades Norwegian music therapy theory, of which I am part. This involves a view of the individual as a unique biological, psychological, aesthetical, and social being with personal resources and rights (Ruud, 2010).

At the same time, the book also resonates with certain philosophical posthumanistic perspectives. These include perspectives that prioritize social actions over individual subjects as those that constitute the individual (Schatzki, 2001). I find the posthumanism perspective that refers to the objectivist practice theory, asserting that social practices include not only humans but also nonhumans (Schatzki, 2001), to be meaningful.

Addressing another person in music therapy improvisation involves engaging in musical actions with that person with a sense of personal commitment. Sometimes this happens with the help of nonhumans, for example, objects with which humans have strong relationships (e.g., musical instruments, smart phones, cuddly toys) (Stensæth, 2013; Stensæth & Eide, 2016; Stensæth & Ruud, 2014). The important aspect is that the actions involved (and their intention, purpose, knowledge, voice) are still those of humans. The concept of responsiveness in music therapy improvisation inspired by Bakhtin's ideas must be understood in this entire complexity.

In my outlining, I will undergo the process of *a reflective synthesis*, which, according to Bruscia (2005, p. 545), involves ...

reflecting on one's own experiences with a phenomenon, relating these to existing ideas or perspectives of other theorists, looking at research, and intuitively synthesizing all these sources of insight into an original theory or vision.

I therefore intend to practice reflexivity, which, again according to Bruscia (2014), requires that I take a meta-perspective not only on relevant theories, but also on myself. I step "out of the ongoing situation for an instant, observe, and then discern what it must look and feel like to all parties involved" (Bruscia, 2014, p. 54). My integration of Bakhtin implies that in my reflexivity, I look more closely at how my ideas lead to a new understanding of responsiveness in music therapy improvisation (cf. Alvesson & Sköldberg, 2000).

To be reflexive, in relation to my treatment of Bakhtin's philosophy—and because I also want the book to be useful in a practical sense, too—I wish to materialize my thoughts empirically by including of a narrative of a music therapy improvisation. I also assume that some of Bakhtin's ideas will emerge from the evolution of the narrative.

THE BOOK'S SCOPE

The scope of the book explores mainly one dimension of music therapy, which is music therapy improvisation. My understanding of the phenomenon is in large part connected to certain traditions within music therapy. These are the Norwegian music therapy community and its perspective on Nordoff-Robbins–oriented improvisation, which I will present shortly. The fact that I am more influenced by this tradition than others makes my reflections and theories even more specific, of course. This means, for example, that because I will speak predominantly from a certain mode of thinking. I cannot therefore speak on behalf of every music therapist. However, since improvisation is a phenomenon that pervades music therapy in various ways, as both a field and a discipline, my reflections may often be general in their scope.

An Indigenous Ideal?

I explore music therapy improvisation from an emic position, from within the phenomenon. I relate, in other words, to a phenomenon that grows out of a particular cultural practice, the experiences deriving from this practice, and the way these are described. It moves from the inside out, so to speak, to make explicit the theoretical and philosophical foundation of its practice.

One might say that it has an "indigenous ideal" (Aigen, 1991, 2005). By indigenous ideal, I mean that my reflections do not always derive directly from the practice of doing music therapy improvisation, but that the aim is to come as close as possible to it. This may also be seen as a way to place my reflections in the middle of the field of music therapy; as Bruscia (2005) puts it, it is *music therapy-centered*:

> It deals with the phenomena as they appear in music therapy settings, as they unfold through music therapy intervention, as they change through music therapy processes, as they make sense within a music therapy context, as they are perceived and languaged by music therapists. (p. 248)

I have tried to obtain the indigenous stance in my reflections by including the music therapy narrative, which is as close as possible as I can come to a practical setting in a book like this, and by referring to myself as the music therapist with an insider perspective.

An Insider Perspective

An insider is one who knows a culture and/or a practice from its inside. He/she has therefore lived experiences and firsthand knowledge about it. By observing myself as a music therapist, I can see the setting from various positions, as both an insider and an outsider. As an insider, I have a privileged access to the knowledge (Kvernbekk, 2005); from within myself and from within a culture of which I am part, I know something that an outsider could not know. This does not mean, however, that I have a more correct or a truer understanding than others. Instead, it means that the insider position is useful for including the more or less immediate experiences connected to music therapy improvisation.

Personal and Professional Context

My interest in the book's topic has several origins. Former studies, personal interests, and clinical experience suggest some of them. Certainly, it would not have been possible to do this study without a personal fascination for music and improvisation as phenomena *and* my professional experience with, and knowledge about, music therapy improvisation as an approach. Therefore, my understanding can be seen in the light of my lived experiences on both a personal and a professional level.

Improvisation has always fascinated me because it involves an attraction to the realms of intuitive and creative activities, especially those involving music. From an early age, I actively participated in musical activities such as singing, playing instruments, and composing music. Yet the greatest joy has always come from doing these activities with other people. Therefore, music and improvisation are, more than anything else, a joint experience for me.

Before graduating as a music therapist, I also studied education and music. During this training, I became aware of my interest in philosophical issues. I realized that I often searched for a connection between improvisation and my life, my music, and my experiences. This can explain my interest in the meta-theoretical aspects of Bakhtin.

Clinical Background

Still, the largest influence on the choice of topic has been my long clinical experience as a music therapist. I can look back on almost 20 years of clinical practice in which music therapy improvisation has represented one of the core approaches. During this time, I have mainly worked in the area of special education with children who have had a variety of needs.

Some children had severe handicaps, while others had minor ones. The severely handicapped children had major, life-threatening challenges; in fact, some of them were so weak that they did not outlive their schooling period. Nevertheless, and despite their various abilities to communicate through words, it was my experience that most of these children often preferred music as a means of communication. In fact, in contrast to some of the large mental and physical challenges, many of them showed a great joy and motivation when being engaged with music. Even if the playing required a lot of energy and struggle, they would still want to play.

This was also the case with Jakob, the client described in the narrative used in the present book. Jakob showed so much vitality and motivation in the music therapy that after a session, he was sweaty and worn out. I often felt so vitalized by his energy, and his absorption with the music and the improvisation inspired me enormously. I learned so much from Jakob, and from everything we shared, just as I have learned from many of the other children and older youth with whom I have worked.

I have seen with many children that the combination of motivation and music creates a potential for therapy in the sense that it enables them to freely express and unfold themselves both mentally and physically. It is also my experience that by being actively engaged in the music, the children cooperate and interact more positively with other people. It is my personal experience that music therapy improvisation helps many children to seek out their own personal resources in order to be able to communicate and unfold. Music therapy improvisation, especially when connected to a phenomenological perspective on human action, therefore contributes to define what music therapy is in relation to many children with special needs.

My Preunderstanding

My preunderstanding, besides the insights obtained from my personal interest and my clinical experience, has two sources. One is the tradition derived from Paul Nordoff and Clive Robbins. This tradition involves an active rather than a receptive approach; it gives greater emphasis to making music rather than to (just) listening to it (Bruscia, 1987; Nordoff & Robbins, 1965). It is a way "to engage the client's attention and diverts inner experiences outward" (Bruscia, 1987, p. 24). In addition, it is seen as a way to keep the client active and interested, as well as a way to "keep the client's emotional experiences in motion, thereby making them accessible to exploration and transformation" (Bruscia, 1987, p. 24; see also Nordoff & Robbins, 1965).

The other source is my master's thesis on music therapy and the phenomenon of play (Stensæth, 2002). This work made me aware of how certain perspectives on play resonate with my thinking about music therapy improvisation. Indeed, I am not the first music therapist to suggest that music therapy improvisation resembles play. Music therapists have already treated the issue. Carolyn Kenny is worth mentioning. In her doctoral thesis, which includes a philosophical elaboration on music therapy, she labels music therapy as "a field of play" (Kenny, 1987/1988, 1989). In my study of play, which was rather different from Kenny's, I was inspired to reconsider my understanding of music therapy improvisation and its relation to the phenomenon of action (Stensæth, 2002, 2008). Action, again, became the crucial point of departure.

This led me to the Norwegian play philosopher, Kjetil Steinsholt, and his descriptions of play (1998). Two aspects in Steinsholt's thinking aroused my interest. One was, as Steinsholt (1998) claims, that play keeps action in the foreground because the motive lies in its content and not in its result.

If one asks children, the real play experts, what they play, they will probably tell you "nothing" or "we just play." They will just play as long as they find their play motivating. When their motivation is lost, they just stop or start playing something else. This, to me, shows how actions, independent of being paradoxical or less rational, are crucial in order for play to be sustained, by suggesting that a strong motivating factor lies in an intrinsic urge to play. I expect this to be true in music therapy improvisation, too. This suggests that we must look for the goal inside the music therapy improvisation, not (only) outside of it—in theories, for example.

The other aspect in Steinsholt's (1998) perspectives on play that I found very interesting is that play "proves" that human beings seek transcendental experiences. Perhaps more than any other phenomenon, play shows how such experiences can be obtained by all of us. This has to do with the way we "lose ourselves" in play and thereby constantly renew our possibilities to act.

I eventually realized that these perspectives on play and its relationship to action resembled Bakhtin's term "carnival," through which the aim is to bring the world close to us through joy and laughter. (I will return to Steinsholt and Bakhtin's carnival in chapter 12.)

A Personal (Musical) Narrative

Behind every theory is a person (Matusov, 2015). Today (and I literally mean today, as I write: February 14, 2017), I realize that one period of time in my life played a particularly significant role for me, my philosophical interests, and my theory-building, both personally and, later, professionally. This was the school year from autumn 1978 to spring 1979 (I turned 15 in October 1978), which I spent at the international boarding school École d'Humanité, located in Hasliberg Goldern, in the Berner Oberland in Switzerland. Because of this sudden understanding, I have chosen to use some space to explain why this period has become an important voice for me.

At the time when I attended École d'Humanité, the school was under the directorship of Natalie Peterson and Armin Lüethi, perhaps two of the most idealistic and inspiring people in my life. The school had been founded in 1934 by the progressive educator Paul Geheeb and his wife, Edith. In 1910, Geheeb had founded a similar school, the Odenwaldschule, in his native Germany. But then he had fled to Switzerland in 1934 to found the new school (which was located in Geneva during the period 1934–1946) after the National Socialists came to power.[3]

The Geheebs were particularly influenced by the German philosopher Ernst Cassirer (1874–1945; in the École d'Humanité, one of the houses was named "Ernst Cassirer Haus"), who was trained in the neo-Kantian Marburg School, a movement that inspired Bakhtin, too (Brandist, 2011). Cassirer developed a theory of symbolism (that later inspired philosopher Suzanne Langer, to whom I will refer to later, in chapter 1) and used it to expand the phenomenology of knowledge into a more general philosophy of culture. In his *Philosophy of Symbolic Forms* (1923–1929), Cassirer argues that man (as he put it in his more popular 1944 book, *Essay on Man*) is a symbolic animal. Cassirer said that whereas animals perceive their world by instincts and direct sensory perception, humans create a universe of symbolic meanings.[4] Cassirer believed that reason's self-realization leads to human liberation and argues that objective and universal validity can be achieved not only in the sciences, but also in practical, cultural, moral, and aesthetic phenomena. These perspectives are in many ways similar to Bakhtin's ideas on the carnival. [Poole (1998) criticizes Bakhtin for not mentioning Cassirer.]

École d'Humanité as a school places a heavy emphasis on the arts, ending academic classes by noon and dedicating the afternoons to all types of arts and crafts, theater, music, dance, and sports. Key elements of the school since its inception have been the absence of grades or required courses and coeducational dormitories for students of all ages. The school motto was in 1978 as it is now: Become Who You Are. The school website describes how they reflect upon their motto today:

> For over a century, these words have expressed the essential challenge that our school invites its students to take on. Moreover, because students are different, this challenge assumes a new form for every one of them. A belief in the utter uniqueness of each student forms the core of the École's philosophy of education. We trust in and respect our students in all their diversity, and we listen to and value their voices.

We foster a culture of individuation and negotiation, a dynamic middle way between conformity and rebellion. École students co-construct their school experience, reflect on their successes and struggles, and find their own particular niches in a cohesive and lively community. Here they are able to grow and express their uniqueness, knowing all the while that they are a necessary and valued part of the whole. In such an environment, they develop confidence in their strengths and aptitudes, a realistic appraisal of their weaknesses and stumbling blocks, and an intrinsic sense of responsibility and compassion. When creative risk is encouraged, education becomes an adventure. (retrieved February 14, 2017, from https://www.ecole.ch/en)

Interestingly, and as I will reflect upon later, many of Bakhtin's ideas resonate with the École's motto. I want to mention one event from that school year. I have come to realize many years later that this event has become particularly significant for me and my life (and my choice of profession). It happened during the singing assembly. The following citation is presented as my personal musical narrative in *Narratives on Musical Life Stories* (Bonde, Ruud, Skånland, & Trondalen, 2013, pp. 347–348):

Karette Stensæth: Every Saturday morning after breakfast, the whole school, including teachers, headmasters, helpers, and students, attended the singing session. One Saturday morning in February 1979 was special. It was right after the tragic death of my father and at a time in my life when I was personally vulnerable and susceptible to emotions. It was also a time when the school board was struggling with problematic behaviour among some of the students. Yet that morning, right after the school had performed a beautiful version of the old (Irish) song "Down in the Sally Gardens," there an unanticipated moment of shared, positive silence. Then, after a few loaded and rather powerful moments, the headmaster at the school, who had just led the singing (while playing his violin), broke the silence with these accurate words: "If we can be together in music this way, everything else becomes easy!" I think that we all felt that this was true. We had been so empowered by the music. In fact, the singing together literally produced a strong feeling of togetherness that encompassed us all, with whatever problems we had at the moment. The program and the École d'Humanité operate under the motto "Become Who Thou Art," and I think that this particular experience in the Saturday singing session explains why I chose to become a music therapist later in life. This community singing not only taught me about the health potential of music but also showed me the broad value of bringing people together and making music, perhaps the easiest and happiest cure for any life challenge. And I have come full circle in this regard; the special education school where I have worked as a music therapist for almost 25 years also offers singing for everyone, every Monday.

One could say, that, just like Bakhtin's "carnival," as I will present later in the book, this condensed event and its context brought the world close to me through its joy, its meaningfulness, and its (serious) laughter. Even today, when I think back on this moment, I experience it again and feel my body shivering from its impact. This event, as well as the whole school year, has made me question whether my interest in Bakhtin's philosophical ideas derives from lived experiences. Have they influenced my theory, too, and if so, how?

The Structure of the Book

The book is divided into 16 chapters, with a Prelude first and a Postlude at the end. Chapter 1 (re)defines central core concepts. (Readers who are acquainted with music therapy theory might want to skip chapter 1.) Chapter 2 describes the phenomenon of action, in depth. Chapters 3–5 involve the music therapy narrative of Jakob and Kaila. Chapters 6–8 introduce Bakhtin and his terminology. In chapters 9–13, I transpose his insight to responsiveness in music therapy improvisation. Chapter 14 presents a theory on music therapy improvisation. In chapters 15 and 16 I will discuss and contextualize the theory.

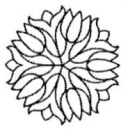

Chapter 1

(Re)Defining Core Concepts

My internalization of Bakhtin's ideas has influenced my understanding of so many terms—not only "responsiveness" and "music therapy," but also "action," "improvisation," "music therapist," and "client," but also terms like "meaning," "time," "aesthetics," and "ethics." To understand where I am going in my theoretical exploration inspired by Bakhtin, I will use some space to (re)define them. The term "ethics" will be presented only briefly in this chapter, to be followed up on in chapters 8–14. The term "action," because it is so crucial in Bakhtin's philosophy, as it is in my understanding of improvisation, is given its own chapter (2).

Responsiveness

What is "responsiveness," and what is typical for responsiveness in music therapy improvisation? The development of this term pervades the whole book, and I will disclose only a few aspects of it at this stage.

Thesaurus.com attributes to "responsiveness" synonyms such as "impracticality," "receptivity," "acceptance," "broad-mindedness," "open-mindedness," and so forth.[5] These are all meaningful in the perspective of music therapy improvisation. Bakhtin's view is more complex and expands the perspective. He claims that there is an inner connection between music as art—or just "art," as he puts it (Bakhtin, 1990)—and life. This inner connection affords responsiveness to others, events, and the world and requires an aesthetic and ethical emphasis.

Bakhtin (1996) then says that a response, to become respons*ive*, insists on action, not in the sense of problem-solving, but in the sense of relating to one another. This responsiveness occurs between people who direct their attention toward each other while actively engaged, face-to-face, in a live situation.

In Bakhtin's picture, responsiveness involves an unfinalized process. Its meaning is not fixed. Rather, it is always at the intersection between the ones who play, between the past and the future of their actions, and between their improvisational event and the world around them. Bakhtin (1984, p. 166) says, "Nothing conclusive has yet taken place in the world, [...] the world is open and free, everything is still in the future and will always be in the future."

Against this background, responsiveness in music therapy improvisation emerges as a situated process and as an enactment of everyday living in music-related terms. It involves, therefore, not just meaningfulness and harmony, but also struggle, dispute, and misunderstandings. Many types of actions might therefore occur—also of the less rational and/or paradoxical kind, or more playlike actions, if one prefers. Such aspects have so far received little attention in the existing theories on music therapy improvisation. This is unfair if one considers music therapy as dealing with the whole range of human actions, including those not understood as turn-taking or as immediately meaningful.

MUSIC THERAPY

What is music therapy? To me as a music therapist, this question is challenging. Bruscia says, "Many music therapists may spend their entire careers trying to find the words to describe their clinical work" (Bruscia, 1987, ix). To respond meaningfully to the question depends upon to whom one is talking. I assume that the people with whom I communicate through this book already have some preunderstanding of what music is and what music therapy could be.

In his 2014 edition of *Defining Music Therapy*, Bruscia says:

> Music therapy is a reflexive process wherein the therapist helps the client to *optimize* the client's health, using various facets of music experience and the relationships formed through them as the impetus for change. As defined here, music therapy is the professional practice component of the discipline, which informs and is informed by theory and research. (p. 36, my italics)

This definition is informative. It includes what I regard to be the main agents in music therapy. These are the client, the music therapist, and the music. Music therapy is also described as a professional and research-based practice. This addition is important for the present book, which is based upon my research elaboration on Bakhtin and how his philosophy may inform and provide new perspectives on music therapy.

During the past 20 years, along with research and theory development within the field, we have seen music therapy develop its own paradigm from within. Such development is, for example, visible in the change of one word in Bruscia's earlier definitions. In the 1989 edition of *Defining Music Therapy*, he says that music therapy is to *achieve* health (as if health is a final goal), whereas in the 1998 edition, he says that music therapy is to *promote* health. This shift, he explains, is done to "signal a complete shift in my ideas about the nature of health; it is a continuum rather than an either-or state" (Bruscia, 1998, xii).

Bruscia then changed the verb again (see the cited definition above). He explains his choice of the word *optimize* as follows:

> To optimize is not merely to improve or to promote; it implies that efforts are made to bring the client to her highest level of becoming healthy, both specifically and generally (p. 40).

I agree with Bruscia that "optimize" is a better word, but I would have preferred saying "a *higher* level of becoming healthy" instead of "her *highest* level ...," because I do not think that there is such a thing as a point in one's life when a person reaches a highest level of becoming healthy. Rather, I see "highest" as an ideal for life, something for which to struggle.

More important is that Bruscia's explanation challenges the role of the therapist. It shows that her role requires a mind-set through which she makes efforts to bring the client to a higher level of becoming healthy.

Dialogues on Music Therapy

Interestingly, before publishing the 2014 edition, Bruscia invited music therapy theorists to join him in a dialogue to redefine music therapy. Bakhtin would have liked this. In fact, for him, the point would be not to end up with a final definition. He would probably have claimed that defining music therapy is, and remains to be, an ongoing and unfinalizable dialogue.

Bakhtin would also claim that as an artistic action, music therapy is most music therapy when it happens in the course of action—it is not defined by the words with which we describe it or the metaphors through which we create images of it.

The Difficult Words

The choice of words is therefore a challenge. When I describe the music therapy narrative in this book and its unique live music experiences, I easily end up with the same words as I have used to describe other very different situations. I therefore might not have enough words or the right words. I have a translation problem: How can I describe the uniqueness of every music therapy situation?

The translation problem is not new. Because music therapists place themselves within many different discursive practices, it is almost impossible to agree upon one unifying descriptive understanding. As Ansdell (1999) suggests, one consequence is that ...

> the "discursive practices" of music therapists become of equal importance to their clinical practices—and should therefore be given equal attention in matters of training, theory-building, and research (p. 14).

I agree with Ansdell in his call for an awareness regarding music therapists' discursive practices. This, however, does not change the articulation problems that we have. Understandably, many music therapists borrow words and terms to define music therapy from other more established theoretical traditions, such as sociology, education, psychology, and so forth. I will borrow mine from Bakhtin.

Eventually, next to emphasizing action, I suggest approaching the question *What is music therapy?* and its answers in the light of its unique situation, its music, actions, and meaning. This suggests a view of music as a phenomenon that consists of sounds primarily characterized through being perceived as signs with meaning (Ruud, 1998). This allows a study of how these signs or sounds are organized, as well as of the social, cultural, biographical, and aesthetical processes that give these signs meaning. It also allows a study of how the music provokes action and inter- or intrapersonal interaction. In turn, this explains how the music becomes meaningful and leads to initiative, change/growth, and health.

Because this book keeps action in the forefront, music therapy orientations that are receptive or those that emphasize and even prefer verbal communication as the main aim of the therapy are left in the background.

HEALTH

The term "health" is complex and broad and involves both mental and physiological aspects. I will delimit my definition of it by referring to Bakhtin and his emphasis on action.

Bakhtin would probably claim that the optimizing of the client's health is a process that is placed outside the therapist and client and inside their actions. I therefore suggest a definition of health as a *capacity for action* [and poor health, a state of suffering or a lack of ability to act (e.g., Nordenfelt, 1991)]. This means that for the therapy to cause growth and change and health optimization, both music therapist and client must first find a common way to act. I therefore sympathize with Bruscia's idea of health as the process of achieving one's fullest (or a "fuller") potential as a human being.

Such an understanding of health also aligns with the old Norwegian understanding of the word "health," "heil," which means whole, uncut, unhurt ("heil, ubeskåren, uskadd"). This perspective originally emphasized health as a state that included an ethical and sociophilosophical way of living, with harmony between body, mind, society, and nature (Schei, 2009). This perspective suggests an existential perspective of health, which I like and which aligns with Bakhtin's dialogical imagination (see chapter 8).

MUSIC THERAPY IMPROVISATION

Inevitably, music therapy improvisation is a large concept in the present book. Considering that it also is a rather broad phenomenon, delimiting is necessary.[6] As many music therapists will agree, music therapy improvisation is also, as process and theory, a way to approach and redefine music therapy itself. The term appears under different names. Some music therapists use the term *clinical improvisation* (Aigen, 1991, 2005; Wigram, 2004), while others use *improvisational music therapy* (Bruscia, 1987; Wigram, 2004). *Music therapy improvisation* is also common (Pavlicevic, 1997, 2000). I prefer "music therapy improvisation" as my terminology. This seems like a better term in the sense that it describes the immediate and main means by which the music therapist improvises and expresses his/her impressions of the situation.

By saying "music therapy improvisation," I think that I point to the aspects that I experience the phenomenon to be about, namely the intertwining of music, therapy, and improvisation. By including music therapy in the label, it is clear that I talk of a particular field. Because improvisation as a phenomenon impresses the phenomenon, it is also important to include improvisation in the term.

I will also link the term directly to the dyad involved in the narrative of this book, where the client is without words and therefore is dependent on the music therapist's ability to engage, interpret, and musicalize his actions and expressions. In the type of therapeutic approach about which I am talking, music and improvisation are close allies. The goals for the music therapy, which I expect to be more or less stable, are many. In fact, all of those mentioned by Bruscia (1998, p. 116) are relevant:

- Establish a nonverbal channel of communication and a bridge to verbal communication
- Provide a fulfilling means of self-expression and identity formation
- Explore various aspects of self in relation to others
- Develop the capacity for interpersonal intimacy
- Develop group skills
- Develop creativity, expressive freedom, and playfulness with various degrees of structure
- Stimulate and develop the senses
- Develop perceptual and cognitive skills

I want to add, however, that any of the above-mentioned goals must be understood in relation to how the musical improvisation becomes a way to deal with the uncertainty of the here-and-now situation through action. According to my experience, this aspect creates an attitude in the client and the music therapist that allows them to take risks and experiment with meaning or, as Ruud suggests, to invest their "fantasies and test other possible ways of being" (Ruud, 1998, p. 179).

Music Therapy Improvisation in the Nordoff-Robbins Tradition

The Nordoff-Robbins approach has had great influence on Norwegian music therapy, of which I am part. I will present their theory in the way that I have personally understood, internalized, and cultivated it.

I find that music and relation, including a clear perception of the role of the music therapist, construct the main concepts in the Nordoff-Robbins approach. Their positioning of the music is one of the core ideas; music is the creative force through which the therapy becomes possible. As Bruscia (1987, p. 24) describes it, the musical improvisation is seen as a "predominant means of interaction and communication between the therapist and the client" and therefore becomes the main crucible for therapy in their approach. Musical parameters like timing, tempo, rhythm, and pauses are the entry points for the music therapist's intervention and interpretation.

Nordoff and Robbins (1971a, p. 16) say that the creation of music becomes the "sphere of experience," out of which the therapy grows. Implied in this image is their assumption that in every child, regardless of ability or disability, lives an inborn musicality and musical sensitivity, which is referred to as the "music child." Several aspects of the Nordoff-Robbins approach can be traced back to the ideas of both Rudolph Steiner, the humanistic anthroposophist, and Abraham Maslow, the humanist psychologist. Bruscia (1987) mentions that ...

> like Steiner, Nordoff and Robbins believed that within every human being there is a musical self which "responds to music, resonates with emotions, and mirrors other aspects of the personality" and "concepts of Maslow found in the Creative Music Therapy include: the channeling of impulses, growth motivation, self-actualisation, intrinsic learning, creativeness, and peak experiences." (p. 68)

Nordoff and Robbins (1977) assert that the "music child" refers to the universality of musical sensitivity, the heritage of complex ...

> sensitivity to the ordering and relationship of tonal and rhythmic movement. It also points to the distinctly personal significance of each child's musical responsiveness (p. 118).

Their assumption that the client's personality is developed from within, using inner resources, does not fit well with Bakhtin's dialogical world. For Bakhtin, nothing, not even the Self, can develop entirely from within, and never without the Other.[7] In fact, a person has no internal sovereign territory but is wholly and always on the boundary, so that when "looking inside himself, he looks into the eyes of another with the eyes of another" (Bakhtin, 1984, p. 287; read more in chapter 8).

What is interesting in the Nordoff-Robbins approach is that their attitude toward the client encompasses a fundamental trust that the music contains many possibilities in which the music therapy improvisation can unfold. For them, this is what creates the needed sphere of experience, which is the basis for the client's growth and well-being. Progression is therefore directly connected to the musical process and the competence of the therapist.

Nordoff and Robbins describe three areas as being the most important:

(1) meeting the child musically,
(2) evoking sound- or music-making responses, and
(3) developing musical skills, expressive freedom, and interresponsiveness.

The areas are illustrated as three work phases in the following model (Bruscia, 1987, p. 45; be aware that Bruscia's model has arrows between the areas).

Figure 1. The Three Work Phases in the Nordoff-Robbins–Oriented Approach.

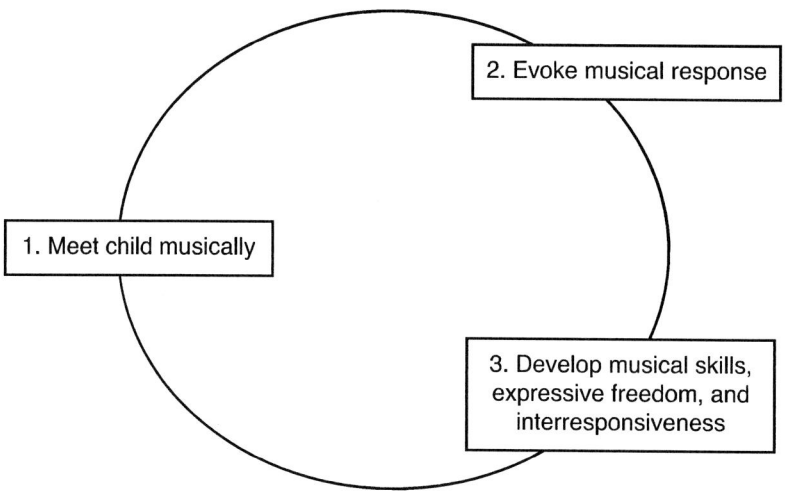

Each work phase is characterized by its own objectives and techniques and is at a different level of development or readiness. The model is not linear, and Bruscia interprets it such that with some clients an entire session or period of therapy may be devoted to one or two phases; with others, a single improvisation may involve all three phases (Bruscia, 1987, p. 44). It is also possible to see the phases and their interrelation as a movement and/or structure of the progression within a single improvisation.

The beginning of an improvisation is perhaps mostly connected to phase one, which is to meet the client musically. Thereafter, there may be more focus on phase two, evoking musical response. Sometimes the improvisation develops toward phase three, developing musical skills, expressive freedom, and interresponsiveness. The third working phase, however, includes the former two, since developing musical skills, expressive freedom, and interresponsiveness alone is not possible to achieve without an intention to meet the child musically and to evoke sound- or music-making responses. In the same way, the second phase predicts the first phase: Evoking sound- or music-making responses is based on meeting the client musically. In the end, the music therapy improvisation turns into a hermeneutic circle in which parts and whole are interrelated and integrated with each other.

This move between phases, parts, and whole necessarily requires a music therapist's ability to move between levels of theorizing in one and the same improvisation. Yet the therapist must not play to express him-/herself, but instead play *clinically*. Rudy Garred (2004), the music therapist and theorist, interprets this as a way to ...

> harmonize with the mood and the emotional level of the client, as perceived in the given situation, rather than trying to play out his or her own feelings there and then (p. 276; Garred refers to Bruscia, 1987, here).

I find that the above citation shows the need for the therapist to be emotionally engaged and aware of the situational differences when meeting with the client.

The second main topic included in the present portrayal of a Nordoff-Robbins–centered theory concerns the relational aspect. From what I both have learned from their writing and seen from their recorded improvisations, the therapist–client relationship is particularly treasured. There is great emphasis on the therapist to express the acceptance, joy, and motivation of being in music as well as making music with the client.

For them, it is important that the client enjoy participating. When his interest and pleasure in the activities increase, the client is motivated to further his expressive musical skills. Nordoff and Robbins also think that every human being deserves to be met as a unique individual in a unique situation. The mix of factors such as personality, time, place, context, interaction history, atmosphere, and so on constructs the setting.

Basically, and as I understand it, it is through the uniqueness of every setting that the musical and relational aspects develop. As we shall see, this emphasizing of action, relation, situation, and joy (or serious laughter, as Bakhtin would name it), mixed with an ethical responsibility (see chapter 11, in particular) to meet each other as unique individuals, resonates well with Bakhtin's ideas as well.

MUSIC THERAPIST

Who is the music therapist?

The fact that many complex areas and practices represent the field of music therapy makes the term "music therapist" challenging to define. Because of manifold practices and professional backgrounds, the role of the music therapist is unclear (Stige, 2015). Ruud says that the difficulties connected to the identification of the music therapist's role have to do with the number of roles he/she has as social worker, special educator, caregiver, and cultural worker. He (Ruud, 1980) concludes:

> In sum, this "trickster" identity not only makes it hard for the public to grasp what professional music therapy is really about, it makes the rules of transaction and interaction and the common basis for a contract upon which to establish any intervention difficult. (p. 147)

Really, the music therapist, as Ruud shows, must negotiate to create a space for intervention in almost every new situation, and often a lot of effort has to be spent on securing boundaries and identities, aiming toward some sort of credibility (Ruud, 1980).

A Supportive Teacher, a Helper, and a Creative Musician

Many labels have nevertheless been suggested to define the music therapist. Nordoff and Robbins talk of the music therapist as a *supportive teacher*, a *helper*, and a *creative musician* (Nordoff & Robbins, 1971a, 1977, 1985). Sometimes, because the therapy process depends upon her being capable of determining the needs of the situation, they almost describe the music therapist *as* the music therapy improvisation.[8] This is visible in the following citation:

> The therapist will find the essence of music therapy to lie in his improvisational creation of music as a language of communication between him and an individual child. The "words" of this language are the components of music at his disposal; its expressive content is carried by his use of them. In the clinical situation, he becomes the centre of musical responsiveness himself; the music his fingers draw from the instrument arises from his impression of the child: facial expression, glance, posture, behaviour, condition—all express that presence his music will reflect and go out to meet. The flexibility of his playing searches out the region of contact and sets the musical ground for interactivity. The timing of his playing—its tempo, its rhythms and pauses—attentively follows, leads, and follows the child's activity. (Nordoff & Robbins, 1971b, pp. 143–144)

A Companion and an Accompanist

Other music therapists define the music therapist differently. Ansdell and Pavlicevic (2005) call the music therapist a *companion* and an *accompanist*. The latter involves not only accompanying the client in sound, but also accompanying the life of the client. This perspective will be reflected in my transferring of Bakhtin's terminology later on.

A "Mother?"

When referring to the influence of theories such as those of Stern (2000) and Malloch and Trevarthen (2009), the music therapist is often compared to the role of a "mother." In particular, it is the mother's caring and instinctive way of relating and attuning to her child that is emphasized in these comparisons. This perspective, because it emphasizes a certain mind-set in the music therapist, is also relevant in this book.

A Participating Observer and a Personal Motivator

We need, however, other foundational characteristics to define the term "music therapist." One is the role of the music therapist as a *participating observer*. The music therapist does not just help, support, accompany, or interpret the client and his musical actions. She also participates and observes the client actively. For instance, to respond and interact empathically toward the client, the music therapist perceives attentively; she sees and listens carefully, whether to musical sounds, verbal language, bodily gestures, or facial expressions, while participating. This requires that the music therapist also is a *personal motivator* for the client.

For Bakhtin, which we shall see in chapter 8, personal and authentic involvement in the Other is essential. Because it belongs to the professional side of being a therapist, it is perhaps odd to require authentic personal involvement. In music therapy improvisation, however, the situation is rather special. My point is that by being actively involved with the musical actions, the music and its aesthetics *stimulate* the music therapist by creating energy, motivation, and pleasure to continue working (authentically) with the client. Therefore, just as she expects the client to be, the music therapist too is energized by the music.

The Music Therapist's Relationship to the Music

Then again, how can the therapist expect the client to be stimulated by the music if she does not experience it herself sometimes? Talking about the role of music in music therapy, Garred says that we need to relate to it as *music*, as an aesthetic force (in contrast to a means for achieving nonmusical goals); if we do not approach it *as* music, we cannot expect any beneficial results to come from it (Garred, 2006). This point, as we shall see in chapter 10, is essential for my transferring of Bakhtin's ideas to music therapy improvisation, too.

The Role of Action in the Music Therapist's Approach

One aspect, which I think identifies the role of the music therapist and also intersects with the book's point of departure, relates to the music as an *action* and *interaction promoter*. To construct a situation through which the musical interactions create a meaningful coherence, the music therapist must often quicken the client to act, which may be a challenge with children who are severely handicapped. Bruscia labels this role as that of an *interactior* (Bruscia, 1996). The term refers to general human interaction and processes such as "matching" and "mirroring," terms that are well known within music therapy improvisation.

My experience is that the role of the music therapist as an interactior is wider than that. Seen from a philosophical perspective, the prefix *inter,* which means "between," is interesting in the sense that the action is seen as something occurring *between* the client and the therapist. The music therapist therefore cannot be seen as being isolated within this task; she also depends upon the client responding to her actions *and* upon the resulting outcome that they together will manage to create something between them. If the music therapist enters the music therapy improvisation with the ideal of relating to the client as a mutual and reciprocal partner, one consequence will be to regard the client as a *co-creator* of his own therapy process.

Summing up the Definition of "Music Therapist"

It seems clear to me that the role of the music therapist, although unclear and difficult to identify with one word, demands several *qualifications*. To sum them up, one might say that successful music therapy improvisation depends upon the music therapist's ability to work musically within the here-and-now together with the client. This requires her managing to work within different mental modalities. Here it is meaningful to mention Bruscia's (2000) call for a move through modes of consciousness. Bruscia suggests here that the therapist in the improvisation does not need to adhere to a particular "perspective" while maintaining the same focus; instead, she must be able to move around in relation to the phenomenon until a more meaningful construction is possible:

> This to me is the essence of therapy, for it is this deconstruction and reconstruction, decontextualizing and recontextualizing, and moving from one mode of consciousness to another that therapist and client do in the process of therapy that lead to more fulfilling meaning as the outcome. Here again, I am saying that meaning is at the center

of both process and outcome, and adding that moving into different modes of consciousness is the key variable. (Bruscia, 2000, p. 90)

I wish to add this perspective here since such mobility within modalities says a great deal about what it really takes for a music therapist to maneuver an improvisation. Bakhtin's theories, and especially his perspectives on the role of the Other, will later add aspects to my definition of the music therapist (cf. chapters 9–11).

CLIENT

Another crucial term is "client." Who is the client, and what role does the client have in the music therapy improvisation?

Obviously, the client is the very reason why the music therapy exists. He is the one who needs help, and it is the client's connection with a problem (which could be more or less articulated) that the therapy seeks to solve.

Client as a Field of Beauty

Yet, in music therapy improvisation, especially when preferring an ecological perspective wherein the client is seen as a whole person with his own personal resources and qualities, "client" is defined within a larger perspective. In her research project, Kenny reminds us that the client and the music therapist are both human beings; each one is a field full of conditions, an environment "similar to the alpine meadow, the swamp, the prairie, and full of beauty, surrounded by beauty" (Kenny, 1989, p. 74). She therefore suggests adding the following image to the definition of client:

> We can say that the client, being a *field of beauty*, is whole and complete, unique, an aesthetic. In a sense, the process of development is to expand this field through increasing certain conditions, or merely re-organizing or creating new patterns of conditions. (Kenny, 1989, my italics)

For me, this image works as an ecological precondition for the music therapist to meet with the client as a (musical) human being with many personal resources. In this sense, the image, romantic as it may seem, reveals that the client becomes the map for the therapy: It is his feelings, expressions, actions, reactions, and responses that inspire the music therapist in her actions and interventions.

This does not mean that the therapist should be blind to the client's difficulties or particular challenges. Without losing sight of beauty and uniqueness, it is just as important to relate to the client's concrete limitations and need for preparation. This is necessary to work toward achievable goals and avoid undesirable development.

Client as Engager

Although the client is not responsible for initiating the music therapy improvisation, it is important to add, albeit implicitly, that the client also has the role of an engager. This is important in order to be able to classify the therapy as serious work (Nordoff & Robbins, 1977).

It also explains why Bruscia characterizes the relationship between the client and the therapist in the Nordoff-Robbins tradition to be a "working relationship" that develops continuously through intense work and participation by both parties (Bruscia, 1987, p. 63). I like Pavlicevic and Ansdell's (2009) distinction between the terms "collaboration" and "communication." They define "collaboration" as "working together" and "communication" as a feeling of sharing and being together.

Client as Collaborator

The client and the therapist collaborate in music therapy improvisation. In fact, just like the therapist's collaboration, the client's collaboration is needed to move the therapy forward. In this sense, the client, to play with Nordoff and Robbins's terminology, also has a role as a serious coworker, just as the therapist does. Their collaboration could give them the feeling of communicating and sharing something meaningful and beautiful. The feeling of sharing occurs on different intensity levels; sometimes it is stronger, sometimes weaker.

MEANING

Therapeutic outcome is often described through the term "meaning," but what is really meant by that term? Meaning occurs when a person experiences meaning. Apparently, however, people experience meaning differently. During my years as a clinician, I have learned that some clients may experience meaning, while others may not. Therefore, to me, meaning is a cloudy concept. I will present those aspects that I believe are most crucial to this book.

Hallgjerd Aksnes and Even Ruud on Meaning

Because it requires both perception and communication, several processes could be considered when we define "meaning." I wish, however, to emphasize those processes that incorporate aspects of music as well as action and interaction, and not purely the verbal aspects. In this sense, I believe that the following definition by Aksnes and Ruud is relevant for the present study:

> By "meaning," we mean simply the conceptualization of something, regardless of whether this something is of a linguistic or nonlinguistic nature. Thus, auditory images, visual and kinaesthetic images, and linguistic associations evoked by sounding music all contribute to the complex network of musical meaning. (Aksnes & Ruud, 2008, p. 6)

Their definition of "meaning" is useful because of their inclusion of the sensory body. For the client who participates in the narrative, this perspective is crucial because he is without words and experiments with meaning through bodily actions. Meaning is not entirely an intellectual process; instead, the body experiences meaning, too, such as through the sensory system.

In the same article, Aksnes and Ruud (2008) also stress that meaning is an *emergent phenomenon*. This aspect is important in improvisation, which is about creating and/or finding significance, or experimenting with intention. One could also say that the meaning is something that emerges through improvising.

The "pre-intentional, nonrepresentational background of shared capacities, practices, and stances toward objects in the world" must be included, too (Aksnes & Ruud, 2008, p. 6). This shows that meaning includes processes of which we are not (yet) aware. Even obvious intentions may be influenced by more or less unknown intentions. This reveals that for the persons participating in music therapy improvisation, meaning includes both conscious and unconscious processes.

Musical Meaning

Also, the music therapist's intention is not necessarily congruent with the intentionality that her music communicates. Composer Bjørn Kruse says that, ideally, the intentionality of the work will coincide with the intention of the artist. This is, however, a "utopian ambition" (Kruse, 2016, p. 43). We must therefore not forget that music is a sensory form among many others, and that the beauty of the music as an art experience is the unique individual interpretation of the participant (read more about Kruse's aesthetics later on in this chapter).

Musical meaning therefore requires musical perception, which creates its own materiality, one that appeals to our senses and our feelings. Perceiving musical meaning in music therapy improvisation is in this way tied to the situation, its culture, style, but also—as we shall soon—its aesthetics.

Meaning as Action

The perspective that meaning, to be expressed, also connects to action is also important. Hence meaning is above all something that the client and the music therapist actively negotiate through their improvisational actions and interactions, whether bodily—through gestures and facial expressions—or musically—through sound and rhythm, and so forth. Therefore, meaning requires actions. It is not something that the client and the therapist passively pass over to one another; rather, it is something that they both actively create together by taking part in it and working with it seriously.

Dialogical Meaning-Making

Matusov (2015, p. 409) says that Bakhtin defined *dialogical meaning-making* as a dialogical relationship between the genuine, personal, authentic question of one person seeking information and the serious reply by another person in a never-ending dialogue. Can we understand meaning in music therapy improvisation similarly? (This question will be explored throughout the book. I will return to it specifically in chapter 16.)

Time

As human beings, we exist in the here-and-now; hence, to act in the world, we need the vital coordinates of time and space.

David Aldridge's Perspective on Chronos and Kairos

Music therapist David Aldridge (2000, 2001) has theorized upon the aspect of action and time in music therapy. According to him, there are two forms of time that are relevant, as defined by the Greeks—*chronos* and *kairos*:

> To act in the world, we need the vital coordinates of time and space. We exist in the now and here [sic.]. While we consider chronological time as important for what we do in terms of coordination, it is the idea of time as *kairos* that is significant. If *chronos* is time as measured, *kairos* is time considered as the right or opportune moment. (Aldridge, 2001, p. 4)

Aldridge (2001) says that to distinguish between time as *chronos* and time as *kairos*, it is the idea of time as *kairos* that is significant. Another way of considering *kairos* is to interpret it as filled time (i.e., the old Greek interpretation). This means that for the event to become kairotic, the participants need to experience time as filled. When the experience relates to meaning of some sort, the time is filled with meaning; it is *meaning-full*.

Musical Time

Aldridge (2001) says that if timing is an ability that is failing, which is often the case with patients with severe brain injuries, then musical form offers an alternative form within which timing can be temporally recovered and practiced, preferably in interaction with others. First, this process demands action in which body and mind are involved, that is, "a creative act of improvising forms of being in time" (Aldridge, 2001, p. 13). Second, it demands a social context because we always seek cognition: "We modify ourselves and others, as they in turn mutually modify us and themselves, through interaction" (Aldridge, 2001, p. 2). Music therapy improvisation, then, is suggested as a way to offer a flexible temporal structure.

This is in line with Abrams (2011), who explains that the temporality in music creates musical time, which affords temporal–

aesthetic doings and interactions. Music, then, offers an alternative form within which timing can be temporarily recovered and practiced. As a result, an experience of coherence and timelessness, something that is typical for kairotic time, is promoted.

Time as Communicative Musicality

Interestingly, Aldridge (1989) views the term "synchronization" as being a core concept in the analysis of the continuous form of communicative processes. To do so, he differentiates between intrapersonal and interpersonal synchronization. This suggests as (1) intrapersonal "self-synchronization" and (2) interpersonal "interactional synchronization" (Aldridge, 1989).

This view resembles that of Ansdell and Pavlicevic (2005), who talk about musicality as a fundamental prototype that "holds together" the mutuality constructed through speaking, moving, and "being with" persons in a social world. This creates a musical community, which is identified through not just time, but also "place." Typically, this creates communicative musicality (Malloch & Trevarthen, 2009), which is typically afforded by music therapy improvisation and its way of establishing togetherness within a setting. This type of "timing" is a premise for the establishment of an intersubjective relationship between a therapist and a client (cf. Trondalen, 2016).

"Participatory Discrepancies"

One aspect I want to mention within the perspective of time is "participatory discrepancies" (Keil, 1995; Keil & Feld, 1994). Discrepancy or variation in good time creates participatory discrepancies, which is typical within genres such as jazz and blues improvisation. The phenomenon, which lies within the music's performance, occurs when there is an intense rhythmic flow and large participation involved in the music-making. When a slight variation in the music happens, such as is the case when playing a little behind the beat (or what is called a "laid back" playing in jazz) or singing "almost" out of tune (sometimes labeled as "blue tones" in the blues), this creates a variation that gives significance to the performance. To recognize the "feel" of the music, one needs to know the culture and be able to participate in it.

Ruud (1998) also believes that participatory discrepancies as a phenomenon are interesting within a music therapy perspective. He explains, "Those experiences that lead to involvement and participation in music originate from a mutual sense of playing around the beat and out of tune" (p. 158). It is also referred to as a "musical discourse around a set of culturally established musical codes," which "emerges in milliseconds and micro-intervals" (p. 158).

Those codes are, however, performed differently in a music therapy improvisation than they are in jazz or blues. The rhythmical flow, for example, may be performed as a *musicalization* (my term) of arm movements or facial gestures, as is shown in connection with the descriptions of the narrative with Jakob and Karla (chapters 4, 5, and 15).

A Place with Groove

Music therapists Gary Ansdell and Mercédès Pavlicevic transfer the idea to music therapy improvisation. They comment that not only do we have to be-in-time-together for successful music therapy improvisation to happen, but also we must "be-in-place-together—where 'place' is somewhere shared and good to be in." Put differently, pulse—the timing of movements and the coherence of such timing—realizes the "place" or the "groove" of the participatory musical community" (both citations are collected from Ansdell & Pavlicevic, 2005, p. 210).

Even Ruud Transposing Victor Turner's "Communitas"

Another aspect that I find interesting within the time perspective concerns the resemblance between liminal experiences and "communitas," which includes a direct, immediate, and total confrontation of identities. I refer here to Ruud's (1998) transferring of communitas, which is a concept introduced by Victor Turner (1969). He refers to communitas as a confrontation of I and Thou in a Buber manner. Communitas is almost always thought of or portrayed by actors as a *timeless* condition, "an eternal now," as "a moment out of time," or as "a state to which the structural view of time is not applicable" (Turner, in Ruud, 1998, p. 132).

Ruud explains that instead of "aesthetic refinement," improvisations in music therapy seek to build such a community through a temporary leveling out of all social roles. Occasionally, when a music therapy improvisation results in liminal experiences of closeness and mutuality between the therapist and the client, such as identified in Turner's communitas, "spontaneous" or "existential" are especially appropriate ways of describing of improvisation. Hence the spirit of community goes before the introduction of rules and social systems (Ruud, 1998). As we shall see in chapters 9–15, such a leveling out of social roles and the existential aspects resemble vital characteristics of Bakhtin's "carnival," too.

"We" in Alfred Schütz's Manner

The last aspect of time is dealt with elsewhere, when Ruud refers to the phenomenological sociologist Alfred Schütz, who treats music as a form of social interaction that precedes verbal communication. This is what Schütz calls the "mutual tuning-in relationship," which originates in the possibility of "living together simultaneously in specific dimensions of time" (Schütz, 1951, p. 78; Schütz, in Ruud, 1998, p. 147). In the "mutual tuning-in relationship," the "I" and the "Thou" are experienced as a "We" by both participants.

Although Schütz refers to the composer and the listener in his presentation on We, it is nevertheless relevant here. It is interesting, for example, to see that Schütz uses the term *inner time* when asserting that the We are lived through in "a simultaneity created by the ongoing flux of experience in 'inner time'" (Schütz, 1951, p. 78). I think this suggests, as does Aldridge (2001) in his theories on synchronization, that both music and interaction are required to identify an experience of We in time-less flow.

Schütz's thinking inspires Ruud to re-view communication, verbal or nonverbal, as socially dependent. Within this perspective, music therapy improvisation is like a miniature of a social system, in which it is possible to construct the tools that the client needs to become involved in a larger social system (Ruud, 1998).

Thus, phenomenologically speaking, says Ruud, the question of *Why music in music therapy?* can be reduced to music's temporal structure and time (Ruud, 1998). I agree with Ruud in his descriptions, which reflect my use of Bakhtin's terms also. (I will return to them in chapters 8–11.)

AESTHETICS

As a term, "aesthetics" refers to sensory perception, that is, the use of senses and/or consciousness. Scientifically, "aesthetics" is often defined as the study of sensory or sensory-emotional values, sometimes described as judgment of sentiment or taste. Interestingly, *an*esthetic, which is the drug that causes anesthesia, is defined as loss of sensation.

In this context, I like to understand aesthetics in this way: as a sense of presence, or the level of presence.

Art as Symbols in Suzanne Langer's View

Susanne K. Langer (1952, 1953/1977) describes in her philosophy of music how music is the tonal analogue of emotive life. Music's function, she emphasizes, is not to stimulate feeling, but to express it. Because the various parts of music have no fixed meaning, we are free to fill its subtle articulate forms with any meaning that fits them. While art forms like painting, sculpture, and architecture create varieties of virtual space, music is different in that it creates virtual time, says Langer (1952, 1953/1977).

This means that time in a piece of music is not understood as the literal time that it takes to hear it or to take part in it, but the virtual time into which the listener/participator enters while hearing it and/or taking part in it. Devices like rhythm, harmonic movement, and many more create the time. Yet most of all it is subjective time—it *is* how each one of us experiences it. Alternatively, even more precisely, what the experience feels like is unique for each one of us.

Langer (1952, 1953/1977) explains that we need music (and art in general) because of the relationship between humans and symbols. As human beings, we need to think and understand through symbols, she says. We also like to "see" a phenomenon through another phenomenon. The power of understanding symbols and regarding sensory data as embodied forms is the most characteristic mental trait of humankind, says Langer (1952, 1953/1977).[9]

Langer refers to two types of symbols: discursive and presentational. Discursive symbolization arranges elements (and not necessarily words) with stable and contextually invariant meanings into a new meaning (Dryden, 2004, on Langer). Presentation symbolization operates independently of elements with fixed and stable meanings. This is primarily experienced and perceived as a whole. The human mind is constantly carrying on a process of symbolic transformation of the experiential data that comes to it, says Langer. She describes symbolism as an unconscious, spontaneous process of abstraction, which goes on all the time in us (Dryden, 2004). Langer (1952, 1953/1977) *therefore* argues that artistic expression and/or rituals are symbols for the experiences and elements of reality, and especially emotional life, which we simply cannot express in verbal language.

Transposed to music therapy improvisation, such as the one between

Jakob and Karla, the client and the therapist in this book's narrative (chapters 3–5), Langer's philosophy suggests that the music therapy improvisation provides forms of experiences other than what words can give them. A single note in the musical arrangement has no fixed meaning for them. Instead, it is the context of the notes and their entire presentation that give her opportunities for gestalt perceptions and opinions that enable them to cross borders in a way that verbal language cannot.

Bjørn Kruse on Dramaturgy and Schiller's Play

When improvising music, the players try to structure a character by "balancing" and creating a certain "level of contrast" between the musical elements. Composer Bjørn Kruse (2016) says that the dynamic interaction of elements such as energy, excitement, intensity, and atmosphere creates the dramaturgical nature of the improvisation. The dramaturgical character of an improvisation relies on the level of detail in focus (from the micro to the macro level). This could refer to how events of interest are experienced as they occur in time and space.

The affordance of the musical improvisation, which is put together by certain elements in a certain way, depends upon someone to appropriate it. The music must first attract someone's attention in order to be experienced as sensory. This requires creative expression and activity through which the performers deal with two simultaneous levels of consciousness: presence in the "now" and a "relative control" over past events and future musical events (Kruse, 2016). The music and its performance are experienced as worthwhile when these events occur in such a way that they hold sustained interest for the person(s) listening to and/or participating in them.

For a person to sustain her interest in the music requires (optimal) balance between two forces, which can also constitute the dialogue between the material tendencies and the will of the player (Kruse, 2016). Through her *willed* action, the performer reveals herself as someone who *wills something*. This will, says Kruse (2016), is akin to philosopher Friedrich Schiller's idea about the three basic human drives: the play drive, the sensuous drive, and the form drive.

Schiller (1967) describes aesthetics as founded on the play drive, which he saw as synonymous with beauty. His *On the Aesthetic Education of Man* celebrates play as a mediating factor that cures humankind's "fragmentation of being" by reconciling reason and nature, form and sense, formal drive and sensual drive, and freedom and necessity. The single most famous sentence in this work is:

Man only plays when he is in the fullest sense of the word a human being, and he is only fully a human being when he plays (Schiller, 1967, p. 107).

Schiller therefore calls the object of the play drive "the living form." Kruse imports Schiller's perception to music and comments:

In the moment of "now" there is a sensuous drive, where the immediate impressions are instantly "chained" to constitute a temporal form through the formal drive, based on the experienced past and the expected future. The third drive is an awareness of the will to acknowledge one's self and intention of being—through a state of playing, or playfulness. The interaction of these three drives is the basic existential dynamism of feeling alive! (Kruse, 2016, p. 65)

A valuation of an aesthetic expression depends, however, on familiarity with the codes in the given culture (cf. Christophersen, 2009). Those who know the musical codes that are used will also appreciate the practice. To define the aesthetics of music in music therapy improvisation, we must first look more closely at the codes used in their way of practicing it. We must also look more closely at the words we use to describe the practice. For example, to what does the aesthetical entity "beautiful" refer, and how does the concrete, bodily, and material practice shape the agents in it? (cf. Ruud, 1996).

In music therapy, the client, and not just the music, becomes an aesthetical *map* for the improvisation (and the therapy). The client is the therapist's music, his score, so to speak. The beauty of the client's feelings, expressions, reactions, and responses guides the music therapist in her improvisation. "Play" and "playfulness," as these terms are presented by Schiller (as drive) and Kruse (as willed action), remind us of Bakhtin's term "carnival," about which we will learn more in chapters 8–11 and 13–14.

ETHICS IN DONALD SCHÖN'S PERSPECTIVE

Music therapy improvisation requires ethical action and reflection by the music therapist. She uses her personal and professional competence, or what Schön (1983) refers to as knowing-in-action. Performing this knowing-in-action requires artistry and ethics, says Schön (1983).

Ethical Artistry

Artistry has dual aspects: One is the art of practical action, which implies the art to implement action so that it turns into interaction. The other is the art of improvising to create a basis for future actions and interactions (Schön, 1983). This part involves ethical considerations and suggests that the music therapist uses individual judgment, at her own discretion. Her professional authority involves, in other words, a responsibility to employ individual discretion and ethical reflection.

Personal judgment normally refers to concepts like tacit knowledge and intuition, a type of ability to judge, but without identifying specifically the kind of knowledge which is in play in the (performance) act. Personal judgment is understood as a supplement to the concrete knowledge, as an added enhancement. Because this type of knowledge is developed through choices of actions based on personal judgment, we may also understand personal judgment as being (a category of and sometimes a "beautification" of) knowledge in and of itself.

Closeness Ethics and/or Situational Ethics

Martinsen (2003, 2005) describes the use of discretion and personal judgment as a type of "closeness ethics" and/or "situational ethics." This requires a common understanding of the situation and that something is experienced as shared. Obviously, the ability to "see" and to interpret the other becomes basic here. I think that the music therapist, when she participates actively and authentically in the here-and-now while seeking knowledge about the client through the musical improvisation, often practices such closeness ethics and/or situational ethics. The music therapist shows her use of discretion and personal judgment through her communicative competence when she, face-to-face, attunes to the client both musically and relationally (Stensæth, 2008). Her interpretation becomes "critical" when she steps out of the immersion of the improvisation to reflect on norms and how to shape future actions (cf. Grimen & Molander, in Tufte, 2011). Bakhtin would frame these ethical aspects within his term "answerability," to which I will return in chapters 8, 10, and 14.

THEORY

What does the term "theory" mean?

Bruscia (2005, p. 540) says, "A theory is a way of thinking about what we do or what we know." Yet, in general, theory is abstract. Kenny suggests that since every new situation brings new and varied elements into our thought structures that are specific to the context, an important goal is to describe the constant elements of our experiences while excluding the unseen structure of our theory (Kenny, 1989).

I think that both Bruscia's definition and Kenny's suggestion are meaningful for the present book. One reveals that theory is personal and around us all the time. The other says that to theorize is to get hold of the constant elements connected to how music therapists describe music therapy improvisation. Both perspectives show that "theory" is a complex term, especially since it is very much connected to a context and the person who constructs it.

To be transparent with regard to the schools of thought that have influenced my thinking, I have defined the most relevant core theoretical concepts. However, because there is a close relationship between theory and practice regarding music therapy improvisation and because both include tacit knowledge and intuition, it is not easy to trace back to the original idea.

Some degree of *introspection* is therefore required (Aigen, 1991, p. 91). To lift my understanding to a surface where it can be tested and evaluated, I look inside myself to understand how I construct my own theory. I also reflect upon what it is about the phenomenon that does or does not receive attention.

From an epistemological point of view, theories are classified differently, and the distinction involves two categories. One is practice-oriented theory. This theory type tells us *how* to practice it, so to speak. Its intention is to realize a meaning, an idea, or a value. In a way, it tends to modify the world. The other category is "pure" theory. This theory type tells us *what* the world looks like. It describes, explains, sometimes preaches, and does not initially intend to modify or realize anything. Many theories on music therapy belong to the first category in the sense that they have a tendency to *guide* practice (Bruscia, 2005).

I assume that my theory in this book is closer to the latter type, "pure" theory. Moreover, I expect it to be useful as a mind-set among music therapists. Hopefully, this will guide music therapists, albeit indirectly, in their doings as well.

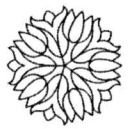

Chapter 2

ACTION

When viewed from the perspective of the phenomenon of responsiveness in music therapy improvisation, the important factor is the idea of the therapist and the client as being actors, co-actors, and inter-actors. With Bakhtin's help, action is kept as a premise for music therapy improvisation and is something that comes *before* collaboration and communication, as stated in this book. This means that action is required from both parties, both the client and the therapist, to realize music therapy improvisation. We therefore need to understand the relationship between the phenomenon of action and music therapy improvisation to understand how the improvisation can optimize health in the client and engage collaboration and communication.

I will begin defining "action" by relating to the sociological perspective. I first refer to Ivar Frønes, the Norwegian sociologist, and George Herbert Mead, the social psychologist. Then I refer to Dag Østerberg, another Norwegian sociologist, who is also a well-known musicologist.[10] I will also refer to Even Ruud, whose definition of music therapy is one of very few, if any, that includes the word "action."

ACTION AND SOCIALIZATION

The term "action" is often explained in connection with the process of socialization. Frønes says that social science theory understands socialization as the external becoming internal (Frønes, 1995). This means that the external world becomes part of the internal, mental world during a process that is known as internalizing. This process often happens unconsciously. Its opposite, externalizing, is about an individual's or group of individuals' influence, energy, and actions. A central sociological point of departure is therefore the relationship between socialization and the acting subject. This involves the development of the acting subject to the psychological "Self."

George Herbert Mead's Social Act

According to George Herbert Mead (1962), the social psychologist, this is constituted as an interaction process between internalizing and externalizing. For Mead, mindfulness arises out of the social act of communication. Thus, the relation between the social process of behavior and the social environment is analogous to the relation between "the individual organism and the physical-biological environment" (Mead, 1962, p. 130).

Mead's concept of the social act is relevant to many facets of social philosophy, as it is for Bakhtin, as we will learn in chapter 8. Mead's view shows how the music therapy improvisation, as a social project between the client and the music therapist, connects to the social relations between the mind, the self, and the society. It also includes the idea that both the client and the music therapist experience the music therapy improvisation within an environment in which these social relations occur.

Ivar Frønes on Socialization

An interesting aspect brought in by Frønes (1995) is that socialization is a problem for the action performer only if it is interpreted as a process of manipulation. Frønes says that in this way, the Self may become too I-weak, so to speak. He suggests, therefore, that socialization is about how the individual is shaped as a unique individual, as a social person, *and* as an action performer. Hence socialization needs to be seen from both perspectives, from the "I" and from the Self (Frønes, 1995).

It seems sensible to add this aspect here, especially when seen from the client's position. It shows that as an individual, a social person, and an action performer, the client, too, and not merely the therapist, influences the music therapy improvisation as both process and meaning. This is basic for Bakhtin, too, who claims that the action is placed between (and almost outside of) the action performers, who approach each other face-to-face (see chapter 8).

Daniel Stern on the Emergent Self

By basing his studies on video-recorded analyses of the relation between mothers and infants, Daniel Stern, the psychiatrist, suggests another perspective on the Self. He believes that the Self emerges through a biologically determined interaction with close others (Stern, 2000). His studies reveal that the infant, to a larger degree than formerly presumed, is more active in his/her own development. The point is that the others with whom the infant interacts are experienced as close. This means that the others' sense and ability to attune empathetically and creatively toward the infant are of large importance in socialization.

This is an important perspective for music therapy improvisation, where the therapy in large part depends on the relation between the client and the music therapist. Many music therapists therefore see a parallel between Stern's ideas and their own thinking. His theories are often applied when they build theories (not least in Trondalen, 2016, and also in Hauge & Tønsberg, 1996, 1998; Holck, 2002, 2004; Trondalen, 2004; Tønsberg & Hauge, 2003).

There are challenges in importing theories such as Stern's, one being that due to the weight of the psychological aspects, the role of action could be left too far in the background. This is not what I want. Rather, with this book I argue that music therapy improvisation depends upon action. As Skårberg suggests, the concept of action keeps the triad of client, music, and therapist together: "Actions are the glue from which musical forms become a net of layers of meaning" (Skårberg, 1998, p. 24, my translation).

"To Increase Possibilities for Action"

Ruud, too, seems to agree with this line of thinking. He includes the concept of action in his theoretical framework for defining music therapy. He claims that what really happens in many music therapy settings is an exchange of actions between people (Ruud, 1998). Thus, music therapy is defined as an effort to "increase possibilities for action" (Ruud, 1998, p. 39).

He continues by explaining that accentuating the concept of action reveals how the music allows both parties in the musical interaction to perform as subjects, taking the initiative and making responses toward each other.

In later works, Ruud (1998, 2010, 2016) uses his definition in a broader social context. His point is that increasing possibilities for action not only involves directing music therapy to the individual needs of clients, trying to empower their developmental skills to increase their personal sense of agency, but also means that because possibilities for action are often hindered by the larger structural barriers in society, there is a need to establish music therapy as something that could meet the broader sociological and cultural needs of the clients (see Ruud, 1998, p. 3). This view requires that the music therapist can see herself as a cultural worker, taking music therapy values and approaches into the community. Later, in chapter 10, we will see that Ruud's view aligns with Bakhtin's call for the ethical responsibility in all of us to approach each other actively and authentically.

My definition of the concept of action within music therapy resembles Ruud's. This view shows above all that "action," both as a phenomenon and a term, is inextricably intertwined with music therapy improvisation. In fact, especially if we keep the narrative used in this book at the center of our attention, it becomes difficult to think of music therapy improvisation *without* thinking of action. Yet, it takes more to describe action than what Ruud's perspective suggests. This has to do with irrational actions.

When I turned to other sociological sources, I found that Østerberg's phenomenological elaborations on action were useful in this regard.

Dag Østerberg on the Phenomenon of Action

Østerberg says that if we are to understand how social life created by human actions and interactions in surroundings is influenced by earlier activity and thereby how a cultural landscape, or a sociomaterial field, is put together, we need first to look at how action as a phenomenon really works (Østerberg, 1993). He suggests that an interpretation of action should be perceived as something other than explaining reasons or causal functional explanations. In contradiction with natural lapses, society does not follow such laws. What happens in society cannot be explained by reasons and sociological legitimations. Ultimately, this makes it impossible to tell what the future will bring.

Actions always unfold within a cultural and/or social field, and in many ways the phenomenon of action defines a human being in that human actions are carriers of meaning, intentions, and transcendence. Deep down, the (ultimate) intention for the human being is to leave a trace behind and be authentic by becoming significant as an individual, toward both him-/herself and others (Østerberg, 2003; Østerberg & Bjørnerheim, 2017).

Action as a Dialectical Phenomenon

Østerberg (1993) explains action as a dialectical phenomenon. (He refers to the nouns "I," "me," and "the other," "him," when he explains this, so I do, too.)

My relationship with the outside world is primarily dialectical, says Østerberg, because my action is dialectical. It is therefore not things in the world, but I who make the relationship dialectical. The other's relationship with me is also dialectical, regardless of myself. Without knowing it, I may be a thing in the other's field of action, but from the moment we both discover each other, we create a mutual dialectical relationship. This is the basis of social interaction:

> What characterizes social interaction is that I treat the other as someone who in turn treats me as one who treats him dialectically. In short, we recognize each other as *acting* individuals (Østerberg, 1993, p. 26, my translation, author's italics).

After discovering each other, we develop greater differences between the unilaterally and mutually dialectic (Østerberg, 1993).

From here, Østerberg divides the phenomenon of action into two types of action, as action-for-me and action-for-the-other. In the first type, action-for-me, the relationship is unilaterally dialectical. In the other type, action-for-the-other, it is different. Østerberg calls this type the mutual dialectical action, which involves both a co-action and a social action.

This type of action gives a signal to the other that the other perceives as a signal. The other's perception of what I have done brings in a new momentum that allows many interpretations. I then might experience the situation and my action as twofold: One thing is what I want to achieve, and another thing is how the other perceives me.

At this point, my encounter with the other has given me an outside perspective and an inside perspective of myself. My mind creates the inside perspective, and my outside perspective is put together by my appearance and my utterances. Then, if I see my own action from the outside perspective, I start seeing myself with the eyes of the other (or the others). From this, we might understand that the mutually dialectical action is the origin of a separation between my actions and my reflections of myself, which is the core of social life.

The Anonymous Action

From this distinction emerges another type of action: the anonymous action. "The anonymous action carries nobody's name; it is every human's action, which has been performed countless times. It is not immediate" (Østerberg, 1993, p. 27). Most of our social life is filled by the anonymous action-for-the-other. This action is formed as duties, orders, conventions, and rituals. The anonymous action is the standardized action that creates a contrast to the authentic action, which is original and spontaneous.

The relationship between the anonymous and authentic spontaneous action is similar to the relationship between action and intention. In a strict sense, we could view action as the unfolding of an intention and as a medium to achieve a goal. In the first, the unfolding of an intention, the purpose of the action is at first unclear. Its purpose emerges throughout the course of the action, but it is only in retrospect that we can see it as an intentional action. When we think, reflect, and theorize, we have already left the action. But our thoughts, reflections, and theories show us the intention behind our actions.

The Unfolding Spontaneous Action

Furthermore, Østerberg (1997) writes that an action that leads to an objectification of the intention reveals the human being for what he or she is. When the actions of many individuals unfold simultaneously, the objectification may be both awkward and distorted. This creates a situation where the individuals do not know in advance in what direction the action is going and that change is possible, maybe also probable. This action we know as socially spontaneous actions that unfold in time within the situation and in the same here-and-now.

This is this type of action that has an improvisational imprint: Its immediacy is oriented toward the future and its intention is (still) indefinite. Østerberg (1993) says that it is through reflection that the action's (past) intention emerges after undergoing a reinterpretation in the light of a changed future. This might sound rather cryptic, but what Østerberg says here is that we understand our intentions in the light of our actions and vice versa. Our reflections are, however, only preliminary results, and the action, because it is spontaneous and improvisational, is therefore prereflective. This action is an unfolding of the spontaneous action. Because it is filled with intentions and also creates new intentions, it remains ambiguous.

This means that the relationship between action and intention cannot be discussed unless they are separated as two different phenomena. In the unfolding of the spontaneous action, intention and action complement each other dialectically. One of them is impossible without the other. This, says Østerberg (1993), excludes an instrumental approach to this type of action.

Actions as a Means for an Intention

An action that is not spontaneous and planned (and therefore is not anonymous) acts differently. Its performance is given. It is unambiguous and serves as a means for an intention that someone had in mind beforehand. This action is a repetition of an intention. When we perform this action, we act in the way it is expected to be done. There is not a dialectical relationship between action and intention here. However, this action is not a total reproduction of a defined intention. Because the situation is new, it is influenced by spontaneity. To put it more precisely: This action presupposes spontaneous action and spontaneous experience.

A Practical View on Action

Østerberg's outlining of action reveals how complex the phenomenon is. His practical view on action shows that it is constantly intertwined with the situation. It shows that action comes first, that the action *is* when it happens within the practical setting. Then follows its interpretation and reflection, which are abstractions of the phenomenon. "Practical" must not be understood as the same as "pragmatic," says Skjervheim (1996). In pragmatic actions, the goal is clear, and their meaning can be scientifically calculated. Practical actions cannot be calculated in the same way. In line with Østerberg, Skjervheim (1996) claims that the aims of practical actions are found in the relationships between people who are communicating with each other in the here-and-now.

I emphasize the word "between" here, because it creates a return to Bakhtin's philosophy (see chapters 8 and 15). To remind you, the reader—and without anticipating Bakhtin's philosophy too much at this point in the book—in his view, action is the origin of his dialogism, which is a complex social and relational event. Bakhtin claims that an action is always on the borderline between the ones who act and between the past and the future of their actions. An action, as a sign filled with meaning, is—to borrow his own words again (Bakhtin, 1981, p. 293)—always "half someone else's" and becomes one's own when it is populated with one's own accent and adapted to one's own semantic and expressive intentions.

THE RELATIONSHIP BETWEEN ACTION AND INTENTION IN MUSIC THERAPY IMPROVISATION

In Østerberg's picture, action contains both the predictable and the unpredictable. This aspect is important for understanding how responsiveness in music therapy improvisation operates.

Action is therefore an equivocal phenomenon, meaning that *an action may realize an intention,* and, at the same time, *an intention may realize the action* (Østerberg, 1993, p. 17, my italics). To me, this explains how an immediate action becomes a realization of something that we do not yet know but which is realized by the action itself, since the intention too is created within the progress of the action. Thus, each action has an intention. However, the intention is neither specific nor defined before the action. In other words, the plan is changed spontaneously. In fact, the plan is both created and shaped on the fly.

Østerberg's explanation clarifies parts of my preunderstanding of the relationship between action and music therapy improvisation; above all, it explains what I have called the "tension" between action and intention. First of all, I find Østerberg's integration of the predictable and the unpredictable into his understanding of the relationship between action and intention especially interesting.

When asserting meanings to be both intentional and non-intentional in different social interactive expressions, such as is done in music therapy improvisation, his grading of intentionality is striking. If we accept that each action has an intention but that the distance between action and intention varies, this could, for instance, suggest that the nonintentional meanings become superfluous (cf. Østerberg, 1993). I therefore suggest drawing an axis between action and intention:

Figure 2. The Action–Intention Axis.

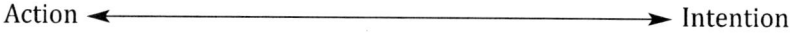

The line connects action and intention and creates a constant and dynamic link, a continuum, between the two. The interesting part, however, is that the arrow goes in both directions. Pointing in one direction, it shows that an action may realize an intention. Pointing in the other direction, it shows that an intention may realize an action. This explains that although there is a constant tension between them, it is not always possible to predict what the action or the intention will end up being.

A constant tension is created between them wherein one is always pushing or pulling the other. Later, in chapter 13, we will see how this axis becomes recognizable within the narrative of the music therapy improvisation with Jakob and Karla. I will also place the image of this all within my use of Bakhtin's ideas in chapter 15, by arguing how this view on action is a premise for responsiveness in music therapy improvisation.

PLAYFUL ACTION

Its glorious mix of pleasure and seriousness, depth and lightness, rationality and nonrationality makes play interesting to anyone who is preoccupied with active improvisation. My experience is that play, and especially its connection to action, relates to music therapy improvisation in ways that are of particular interest to the topic of the present book. This refers again to what in the Introduction I called the less rational and/or paradoxical aspects of the relationship between music therapy improvisation and action, a view that also reflects Bakhtin's term "carnival" (see chapter 8).

To understand the character of play, we need only to watch children entangled in play: One can literally see inspiration and contentment in their faces as the children lose themselves in play. While playing, children reveal great joy and satisfaction coupled with a strong sense of presence, as if the world outside of play is nonexistent. Also, one sees that the children seek optimal inspiration and contentment through their aesthetic creative being and doing by changing the rules and directions of their playing every other second (or so it would seem).

This could show how the individual, as he/she is so strongly inspired, is willing to stretch his/her mental and physical capacity, sometimes even to its very limit. Inspiration and contentment are characteristic aspects of the phenomenon of play; together, they create another playlike aspect.

Several theorists, including many music therapy theorists, claim along with me that the phenomenon of play is a good model for understanding the construction of improvisation and creative aesthetic actions (Csikszentmihalyi, 1990; Gadamer, 2003; Holck, 2004; Kenny, 2005; Leontjev, 1977; Pavlicevic, 2002; Steinsholt, 1998; Tønsberg & Hauge, 2003). I will include small but central aspects of the theories of Leontjev and Csikszentmihalyi.

Aleksei Leontjev on Play

The Russian psychologist Aleksei Leontjev (1977) claims that play works through conflict between two central components: the need to act and the way to perform the action. Leontjev suggests that only play manages to solve this conflict because the motif lies in the *action as content* and not as result. Without saying that the music therapy improvisation is without goals or intentions, this made me realize that by allowing actions to create the forefront, one consequence is that all actions, including the less rational, are of great importance.

Mihaly Csikszentmihalyi on Action Possibilities and Challenges

Mihaly Csikszentmihalyi's (1990) perspective on flow is interesting in this respect. He uses the term "flow" to describe this state of mind in which a person feels intense inspiration and contentment. During moments of (constructive) flow, a person is highly creative and activity becomes simple and effortless. I am not especially interested in the flow experience as such. I am interested in the way in which Csikszentmihalyi discusses flow in relation to two dimensions: (1) the individual's action possibilities and action challenges, and (2) the individual's capability and opportunity to act.

The first dimension involves natural external impetus, such as food, nature, and social environment, while the second relates to internal impetus, such as motivation, mental capacity, and learning. Included in both dimensions is action competence. Therefore, to realize the process *toward* flow, actions are required. This process is very much impressed by a strong feeling of presence, which is also characteristic to play and other creative and aesthetic activities.

A SHORT SUMMING UP ON ACTION

Action—preferably as a dialectic, social, spontaneous, playful, and risk-tempting phenomenon—is required to achieve inspiration and contentment, which could lead to transcendent experiences. This in turn is vital to the understanding of how music therapy improvisation might engage client and therapist in responsiveness with the potential to create meaning and optimize health.

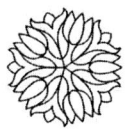

Chapter 3

INTRODUCING THE MUSIC THERAPY NARRATIVE

This chapter presents the narrative that is meant to serve as an exemplar of music therapy improvisation that represents a perspective—a plea—in the discussion of my implementation of Bakhtin's ideas.

The narrative involves two people: Jakob, the client, and his music therapist, me, whom I will call Karla. Jakob and I had music therapy together for seven years in the special education school that he attended and where I worked when the music therapy improvisation took place. We knew each other well as improvising musicians, and we both knew what to expect from each other.[11]

Our improvisation was arranged for my PhD thesis (Stensæth, 2008), in which the data collection process, including the observations on the video recording and its analysis, is described in detail. This book refers to two excerpts (three minutes) of the video-recorded improvisation. One excerpt is called The Guitar Excerpt, and the other, The Djembe Excerpt. I have attached the scores of the excerpts in the back of the book. Its function is mainly as a map. The narrative is based on qualitative observations, logs, and analyses of these two excerpts.

THE OBSERVATIONS

The observations were made by 11 experienced music therapists. One of the observations was made by me.

Indirectly, the observations mediate between the "inner world of the participants' thought-feeling and an outer world of observable actions and states of affairs" that were visible on the video recording (Kenny, 2005, p. 116; Kenny quotes Bruner here). The observations create associations to old "field notes" and an aspect of autoethnography, which is a method in narrative inquiry that situates the researcher within the context of the culture being studied. The researcher tells his or her own story as an insider.

As field notes, they appear as descriptive observations of a setting and an event involving people from the "tribal society" (the music therapists). The observers' voices operate as the voices of insiders, "providing an important emic position within, and therefore creating trust in the teller, diminishing the problems of representation from the outside" (Kenny, 2005, p. 418).

Although the 10 other observers did not participate in the live setting as I did, they were indirectly situated (that is, by observing a video-recorded example of a situation with which all of them were familiar). Eventually, these perspectives support the indigenous ideal, which I have already stated as a lodestar in this book project.

Differences between My Observation and the Other Observations

My own observation is different from the other observations in several ways. One is the amount of attention given to the music. The weight is different in my observation, where the musical aspects have been thoroughly systemized and in which the rhythmical aspects, whether through playing the instrument or vocalizing, are accentuated as particularly salient in the interaction.

The other observations do not include many details about the sound and the music. Paradoxically, it is not so much the music, but rather the absence of music (e.g., breaks, pauses, spaces) that has largely been described as "created," for example, to give room for the other player in the interaction to make his/her move.

Another tendency is that the other observers, because of an immediate fascination with the client's manifest engagement and spirit, tend to slightly overrate his abilities. For instance, it is noted that because he often tops off a musical line, he has a well-developed sense of musical phrasing, whereas in my observation it is suggested that his fragmentary utterances reveal his way of playing and vocalizing, meaning by this that he can act only through short phrases, one at a time.

It is suggested in my observation that the client, because of his personal style and his great enthusiasm for music, possibly experiences the musical interaction so strongly that he actually needs to withdraw every once in a while, to collect himself.

Where it concerns the client's arm movements, which have received a lot of attention from all 11 observers (including me), it is mainly in my observation that it is defined as a part of his bodily sensory reaction, which comes spontaneously as he is stimulated by the music. The other observers tend to interpret his arm movements as consciously intended.

A reasonable conclusion of the comparison between my observation and the other 10 observations is that despite the differences and because of the large consensus between the observations and my analysis, the observations officiate as validation of my own observation. I therefore find it useful to create one narrative of all observations for the present book.

The Logs

My use of logs appears to be rather personal, something that probably relates to the fact that they were expressed by me, the music therapist, from within the real setting.

The language in the logs came out differently, as it involved feelings, comments, images, and/or thoughts that came into my mind as a music therapist within the setting. Single words, metaphors, drawings and illustrations, and so on were typical for this language, which created a fragmented result and a somewhat "poetic" tone.

From another perspective, this time from that of the observing music therapist, another type of language was required, one that was of a less personal type than that used in the logs. Whereas I was actually present as the actions took place and the music therapy improvisation was being shaped, as an observer I was at a distanced position. Obviously, I could no longer change or influence the course of action; rather, I could step back and try to understand why and how the actions took place (there and then), while at the same time being aware that indirectly I carried with me the spirit of the live situation.

The Image of Michelangelo's Creation of Adam

At some places in the logs, when I have written down just one word or done a drawing, I have filled out the story behind it. Usually, this story connected to an image that was familiar to me in the sense that it came to my mind in an earlier music therapy improvisation, either with this client or in other settings with other clients.

One of these images was, for example, Michelangelo's *Creation of Adam*, which was originally painted on the ceiling of the Sistine Chapel in Rome's St. Peter's Cathedral. This image popped into my mind as a music therapist during the music therapy improvisation with Jakob. When I drew two fingers pointing at each other in the logs, I was trying to describe that I had experienced something in the improvisation of which Michelangelo's *Creation of Adam* was a good illustration.

The drawing indicated that I, as the music therapist, had experienced that Jakob and I were reaching out to each other and that we *almost* touched. At the same time, I experienced stepping "outside" the course of action for a moment and seeing the client and myself in the music therapy improvisation from another level (from the "ceiling" perspective, perhaps). When I drew the pointing fingers in the logs, I "knew" the story and thus I did not have to explain the experience fully there.

Challenges Connected to my Merging of the Observations into one Narrative

The main challenge connected to the treatment of the observations and the logs did not concern the variations in the observers' stories or the fact that the observers represented different contexts. Instead, it was connected to my presentation of them: How could I, as the author of the text, tell the observers' stories without disturbing their voices too much?

Eventually, I found that it turned into a question of authenticity and trustworthiness, aspects which seemed to be best maintained by letting each participant use his/her own voice as much as possible in the telling of his/her story concerning experiencing the video-recorded excerpt. I decided to refer to them as "the observers." Sometimes, when the observers had made a particularly good or striking description, I cited these.

All in all, I feel that the narrative portrays the observers' voices with a degree of neutrality and authenticity. I believe that reflexivity in my elaboration is still possible to maintain, as I can subsequently allow parts of the observations to interact with my own interpretations when I mix them with the theoretical and philosophical aspects at a later stage in the elaboration.

After all, the main concern at this stage of the book is to create an intersubjective space, which in turn can initiate a meaningful dialogue around the aspects that I am tracing.

I have decided to regard the elaboration as interplay between several crucial parties involved in my own theory on music therapy improvisation, as a polyphonic texture of syntactical, semantic, and pragmatic meanings that is an important aspect of any functioning, experiential work (Ferrara, 1984).

How to Read the Narrative

The narrative should not be read as a neutral story. It is a version of an event, which is my interpretation, which in turn is inflected by many voices from many people, theories, and cultures. These voices are not passive. I align myself with Blaikie (2003), who says that if we relate to observations only as passive objects or events waiting to be coded or granted shape and significance through our interpretative work, they turn into tools through which we arrive at a (research) conclusion.

I do not want to end up with a conclusion or a final story of the music therapy improvisation between Jakob and Karla. I am aware that the narrative includes much more than what I have been able to see or what you, the reader, can read from it in a book like this. Because I am a researcher and a music therapist, my mandates unite in the need to observe and to interpret, but I know that the narrative hides unexpected appearances and "secrets," which you or I are not able to see (yet).

As Bakhtin put it, as a human being living in a world with other human beings, I can face the world actively only by directing my attention toward others (either clients or you readers). However, by being aware of the potentially hidden aspects in the narrative, I might be more open toward such aspects, too. In this way, I might find aspects that Bakhtin emphasizes in his dialogical universe (see chapter 8), which are those aspects that are easily misunderstood and which do not immediately make sense.

In order to delimit the details of the data material for a book like this, I have tried to collect those aspects in the narrative that I find sufficient to illustrate my internalization of Bakhtin's ideas.

The Structure of the Narrative

The narrative will be presented with a mix of the various data (observations of the video-recorded improvisation, logs written by the music therapist from within the natural setting, observations and scores of the video-recorded improvisation).

I will first present the descriptions of The Guitar Excerpt. Then follow the descriptions of The Djembe Excerpt. The Djembe Excerpt is longer than The Guitar Excerpt, a fact that is reflected in the relative lengths of the descriptions of these two excerpts. I sum up descriptions of both excerpts at the end of the narrative.

The narrative is written as a whole and starts with a section that is seen mostly from the perspective of Karla. Then follow sections in which the voices of all 11 observers are merged. Aspects from the logs and the scores of the improvisation are used to complement the descriptions.

The parts that involve Karla's images and her self-dialogue are indented in the text.

For the sake of communication and clarity, I will refer to the different voices connected to my roles (as a music therapist within the setting and as an observer of the video recording of the setting) in the third person throughout the narrative—as *Karla* and/or *the music therapist*.

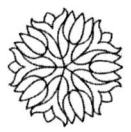

Chapter 4

THE NARRATIVE OF JAKOB AND KARLA

Karla hears some familiar sounds from the hallway as she prepares the music room for the music therapy session. It is Jakob gurgling cheerfully as his caretaker wheels him toward the music room in his wheelchair. Karla notices that hearing these sounds makes her smile. The sound of him enthuses her, and his cheerfulness is contagious. At the same time, she realizes that several images pop up in her head, like flashes of feelings.

Karla "sees" Jakob: all of him. She sees the slim body in the wheelchair, his face with this expectant, interrogative, and slightly frightened look, his arms moving in all directions, and how he suddenly crosses them every once in a while, and she sees the center of his body making small shaking movements. She remembers how she perceives his sounds and his body as one expression, an expression that is somewhat chaotic, but full of spirit—always ready to move somewhere musically, always ready for the next step! A question (which she remembers has come to her before) emerges: Is this his surplus of energy and action that cries to come out?

Then Jakob turns up in the doorway along with his caretaker ...

THE GUITAR EXCERPT

Karla and Jakob face each other. Karla directs her face, body, and the guitar toward him, as if inviting Jakob to play with her. She begins by stroking the guitar strings gently on the first beat.

Figure 3. Rhythmical Development in the Therapist's Guitar-Playing.

Bars 1–2 in The Guitar Excerpt

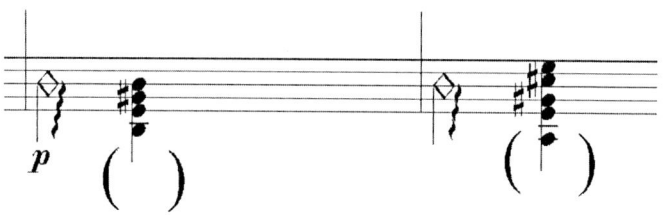

Then she introduces a steadier, "swinging" rhythm.

Figure 4. Swinging Rhythm in the Guitar-Playing.

Bars 4–5 in The Guitar Excerpt

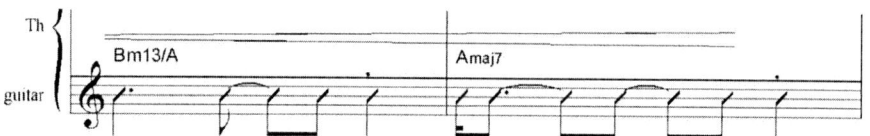

There is a pattern in the sense of rhythmical development in the way that Karla uses her right hand on the guitar. She seems to try to set a mood, an agenda, by stabilizing a tonal center and inviting Jakob to join in. She varies the rhythms again by adjusting to the way she sings.

Figure 5. Varying the Guitar Rhythm.

Bars 10–11 in The Guitar Excerpt

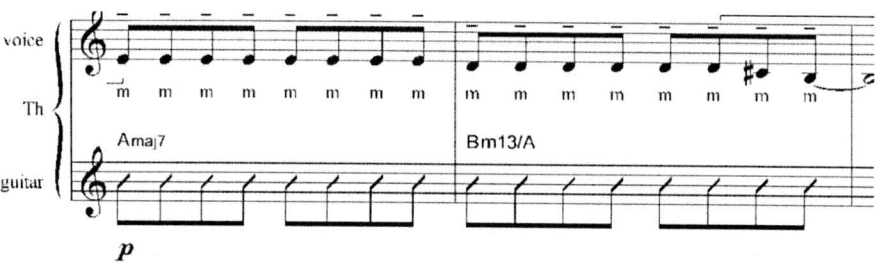

To include Jakob in the music therapy improvisation, Karla uses several techniques. As in a mother–infant relationship, she interprets his arm gestures as musical initiatives or responses—acting as a mother would. This is probably not something of which Jakob is aware (yet). For him, gestures and bodily expressions are still his natural and intuitive way of unfolding and expressing himself, and thus his arm movements probably reflect Karla's music directly.

Still, there is a chance that Jakob experiences (unconsciously) that his reactions and movements also influence Karla's music. For example, it could be that Jakob experiences Karla's vocalizing, as exemplified above (bars 10 and 11 in the score), as a statement and a question directed toward him, saying something like: "I [Karla] hear what you say and how you express it. Can you hear me doing something similar to what you are doing? In fact, can you hear what you yourself say and how you express yourself when I reflect your way of doing this?"

From this perspective, the musical improvisation is sometimes treated as questions between Jakob and Karla, as if there is actually a verbal dialogue going on.

Jakob listens to Karla in a calm and collected way. His hands are relaxed. He keeps a posture in which he is turned toward the guitar and Karla's playing as if wondering: "What is happening here?" Her singing catches his attention. It is as if he questions himself: "Doesn't her music sound 'familiar'?" "Do I hear [or am I imagining] that she is imitating me and my voice and my way of singing?"

An image immediately pops into Karla's head—the image of a café:

> Karla finds herself standing outside the café looking through the window. On the inside, she sees two people drinking their lattes. They are turned toward each other—and focus their attention by asking: How are you ...? How are we ...? What shall we talk about? How shall we talk? They seem to have a lively conversation; their faces are expressive, alternately smiling and raising their eyebrows. They really make a lot of gestures, and one of them moves his arms a lot (Is he making some sort of a statement?). They are intensely present, but she wonders how well they really know each other. [...] The coffee drinking seems to create a shape between them so that they know what to do with their hands. When one of them raises his/her cup, the other follows suit. The movements create a center between the two of them—.

> *Karla starts thinking about this "center" as she plays the guitar. The center seems to create a frame that outlines an invisible crucible of the interaction space that is between the two of them. The space seems magic in some way, as if it is magnetic for Jakob. "Is it magnetic for me, too?," Karla wonders.*

Suddenly, Karla becomes aware that her thoughts are drifting away, partly away from Jakob. She tries to refocus entirely on him: She hears his voice, his stutter-like utterances, as if he is clearing his voice and preparing himself to say something, something important. But she cannot really hear what he says, and she realizes that she would have liked to hear what he wants to say. Then she realizes that he actually says something to her. Karla questions herself: "Does he [Jakob] ask me about something? Or does he invite me to join him in the framing of the questions?"

> *Karla then sees Jakob's face, an open face, a pleased but expecting face, an expressive and slightly worried face, his big brown eyes that never really look right into her eyes, and she realizes that she wants to make eye contact with him. Although she is aware that this is how he always uses his eyes, this makes her feel uncertain. She questions whether he might use his eyes in the way he uses his sensory apparatus, always wandering around, first toward the guitar and the playing, then away from the guitar and the playing, and then back to the guitar and then toward the center of the space that is between them ...*

The bass note coming from the low A-string on the guitar imprints their improvisation so far. This note sounds as a pedal point and creates a tonal center of A major. The fact that Karla plays various chords and changes her rhythmical playing does not disturb this impression.

In the final bars, she intensifies the rhythm by playing faster and ff.

Figure 6. Playing Faster ...

Bars 25–29 in The Guitar Excerpt

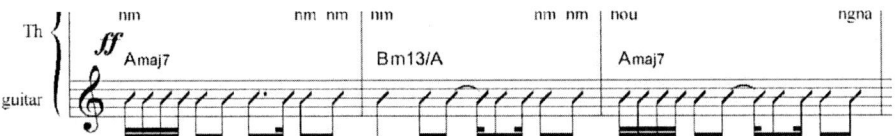

During *The Guitar Excerpt*, the music gets the character of a prelude in the sense that the Karla tries to set a mood, an agenda, by stabilizing a tonal center and inviting Jakob to join in.

By looking at the scores only, it seems obvious that in a musical sense, it is Karla who is the most active participant; she both plays the guitar and sings, while Jakob makes only sporadic vocal utterances. However, this picture changes when the video excerpt is observed, as this reveals how active Jakob really is—in a bodily sense, that is. He moves his arms a lot, crosses them, and lifts them up into the air.

She often directs her face, body, and the guitar toward him, as if inviting him to play with her.

The vocalizing colors *The Guitar Excerpt*: Jakob's vocalizing is mostly staccato-like singing utterances, while Karla varies her vocalizing more. (In bar 13 of the scores, it sounds as if Karla vocalizes in a way similar to that of Jakob.) Additionally, there seems to be a pattern in the use of pauses, something that Karla seems to initiate: When Jakob vocalizes, Karla either stops her rhythmical guitar-playing or "rests" her singing on a long tone (see, e.g., bars 9, 12, and 24 in the scores). She also "sings" long notes in other places (bars 8, 9, 12, 18, 19, 20, and 21 in the scores). Additionally, she uses upbeats a lot, first with the guitar (bar 3) and then with her voice (see bars 19, 20, 23, 25, and 26 in the scores).

> Karla becomes aware of her own feelings, that it is time for her to move on, that it seems impossible for her to stay any longer within this intense mode, and that she needs air—She needs to "breathe." Doesn't he need to "breathe," too ...?

> Karla also becomes aware of her own pushing and thinks: "Is this too much for him?" "Can I go further?" She wonders if she is being too intervening, too "invading." Yet she senses that he

is safe, that he knows what to expect, and she finds that it is time to open up and to offer him an instrument ...

The impression given is that Karla challenges Jakob, for instance, by testing out how much musical stimulus he desires. This indicates that there is an established relationship between the two of them and that both of them feel safe in the interaction. There is also reason to believe that an inspired Jakob challenges Karla, or at least it seems as if this is the case from the way she develops her music and alternately plays loud and soft strokes on the guitar to continue stimulating the client (see bars 21–24 in the scores of The Guitar Excerpt).

THE DJEMBE EXCERPT

Later on, in The Djembe Excerpt, the setting is changed, as Jakob and Karla play on the same instrument. They take turns in beating the djembe, and each creates small announcements and phrases directed toward the other.

The fact that only one of the parties can play at any one time is perhaps the reason why there is a rather salient musical interaction going on in this part of the improvisation, an interaction that mainly involves an exchange of small rhythmical patterns. (Naturally, they can both vocalize independently of each other and their drum-playing.) Another reason is perhaps the fact that there is always a little space/time before each initiative, something that isolates the musical announcements. This is marked in the scores with dotted lines, for example, as in the beginning of the excerpt.

Figure 7. Exchange of Rhythm.

No. 1 in The Djembe Excerpt

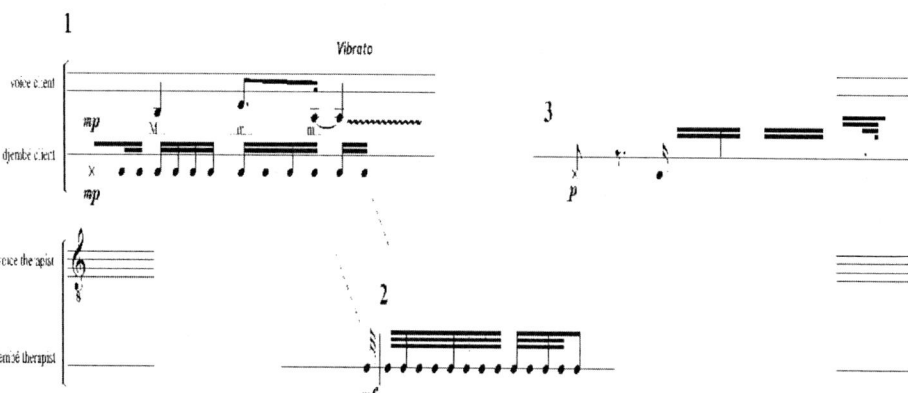

There is one section in this excerpt that differs from the isolated phrasing (like the one in Figure 7), and this starts at no. 7 and lasts until no. 13 in the scores. This section, which has already touched upon, involves longer phrasing and develops musically in terms of musical complexity. Here one can see a longer interaction phrase starting.

Figure 8. Longer Interaction Phrase.

Nos. 7–8 in The Djembe Excerpt

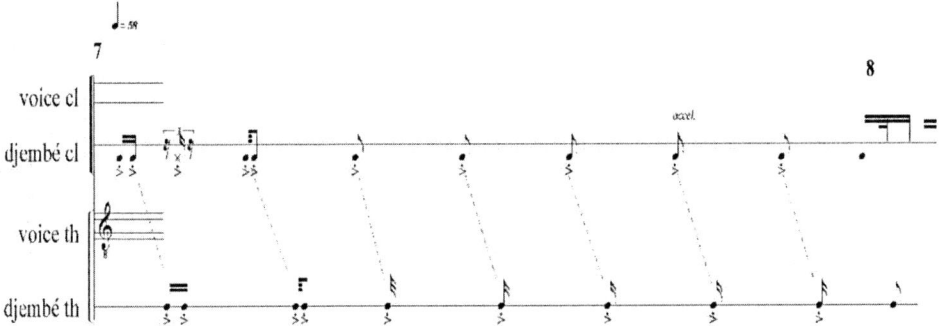

The impression here is not that the musical announcements are isolated, but rather that together they create a whole. (In fact, it is not easy to tell from the sound who plays what, or who takes the initiative and who responds. This explains why the music lines are connected in this part of the scores.)

However, a variation is recognizable in the way the drumbeats sound, and by looking at the scores, one can see that Jakob (cl) uses a little longer time (space) before he comes with his initiatives. Additionally, his beats last a little longer than Karla's (th) beats. It feels as if this individual way of beating the djembe creates one type of dynamic.

Another type is Jakob's use of space before beating. Both create a delayed synchronicity, which again increases the intensity in this part of the improvisation.

At no. 8 in the scores of this excerpt, the sound of Jakob's scratching on the drum skin creates a musical uncertainty, and for a short while it is doubtful whether the music will continue to develop. Interestingly however, the musical interaction continues with powerful strength and greater complexity in no. 9 in the scores.

Figure 9. Powerful Strength and Greater Complexity.

Nos. 9–12 in The Djembe Excerpt

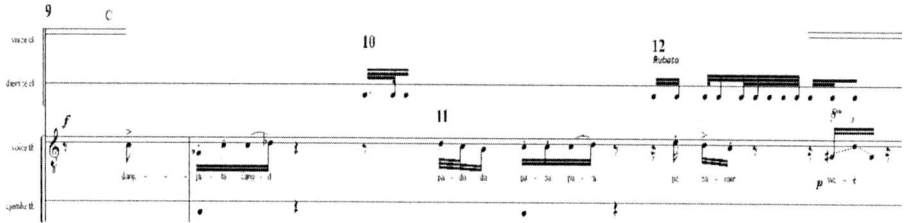

First, Karla (th) introduces her voice (no. 9 in the scores). She vocalizes a melodic pattern whereby she accompanies herself by playing the djembe on the first beat of each motif. Then there is a silence.

The three "hasty" beats at no. 10 in the scores made by Jakob (cl) sound like a follow-up of what has just been described. In no. 11 in the scores, it sounds as Karla briefly vocalizes Jakob's djembe-playing (in no. 10 in the scores) before she continues to vocalize and accompany herself again (similar to what she initially did at no. 9 in the scores).

After a short silence, Jakob starts beating the djembe more actively, and now Karla starts to accompany his playing by vocalizing. The development dies out during nos. 13 and 14 in the scores, as one of the active parties (Jakob) is absent in the musical interaction.

Still, there are other places in the excerpt in which one accompanies the other (for the main part, Karla accompanies Jakob). This kind of interaction is, for instance, recognizable at no. 26, at the end of the excerpt.

Figure 10. Karla Accompanies Jakob.

No. 26 in The Djembe Excerpt

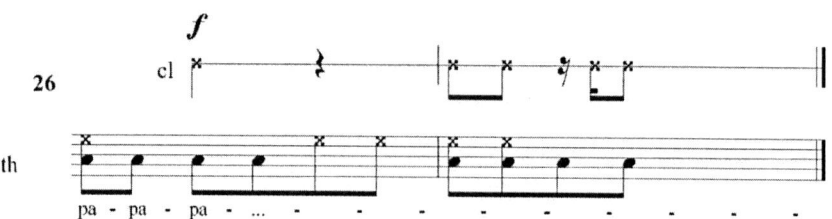

In contrast to the delayed synchronicity, which we saw in nos. 7 and 8 in the scores, which was obvious in the former music example, this example involves a "perfect" timing in the interaction, especially in the last bar, where Jakob and Karla twice beat the djembe simultaneously.

The Djembe Excerpt is a working phase in the music therapy improvisation that is clearly organized. This may be due to more focused attention from both participants and the simple setting in which the two of them surround one instrument and face each other directly, something which provides a better overview for both of them with regard to what to do and how to do it.

This also explains Jakob's apparently skilled interaction in parts of this excerpt: He is in a position where he can observe and interpret Karla's actions precisely, and, as only one of them plays at any one time, the turn-taking becomes more evidential for him.

The excerpt is characterized by interaction, as if there is a musical and a relational negotiation going on. Here the actions seem to be more directed onto the person sitting opposite, in contrast to the former excerpt.

For Jakob, the interaction perhaps stretched him to his limit, in terms of both developmental capacity and energy. The impression is given that Karla consciously challenges Jakob a great deal and in a more direct way in this part of the music therapy improvisation than is visible in the previous excerpt. It is as if she explores how far she can go musically to challenge him, that is, to find out how much sound he can bear, how fast he likes her to play, and how long a phrase she can play while he listens with interest.

No. 4 in the scores of The Djembe Excerpt is an example of this, because obviously, she is aware that Jakob is not capable of playing something similar when she makes the long and rather "advanced" phrase on the djembe. It is fascinating to see Jakob's reactions afterward, because it is evident that Karla's challenge does not lose him; instead, it seems as though her move increases his engagement in the interaction and brings his consciousness to another level.

Karla questions herself: Is Jakob challenged?! He seems interested but unsure—as if he does not know what to expect from her, how loud she will play or how intense she will be. Does he quicken? Does he accept her pushing?

Jakob then keeps his arms "indecisively" in the air, as if he does not know where to put them. He "sings" by humming on "hm hm hm" and then *raises his arms way up in the air as if joining the dance ... (a flamenco dance?).*

Karla starts to wonder: Does Jakob imitate my rapid playing, or ...?

At first, Jakob reacts bodily by crossing his arms high up three times. (In one observation, it is also noted that he "listens, actively, as if he needs to 'digest' what the music therapist is doing.")

Jakob crosses arms again but not as tightly as before, withdraws a little, crosses arms ... as if negotiating with himself ("Shall I let go—or shan't I?")

Then, it seems as if he tries to come up with something similar to hers. He makes a vocal sound and prepares his right hand for some playing—makes some more vocal sounds (staccato)—makes a movement as if playing a drum in the air with his right hand before moving it down and hitting the djembe—plays rapidly and distinctly (f).

It is possible that Karla's almost provocative challenging of Jakob induces a small breakthrough in that the music therapy interaction moves into a more salient and apparently conscious turn-taking (around no. 7 in the scores).

However, it could be that this interpretation is too benevolent and that Karla's challenging attitude is too much for Jakob. For example, her voice is described in one observation as being too "near" and too "strong" for him at around no. 10 in the scores. This indicates perhaps that there must be a trusting relationship between them, because, evidently, Karla's actions balance between fruitful and too much. In this sense, she relates to the music therapy improvisation as a way to explore him and his capabilities, whether actions, concentration, interest, or so on.

Interestingly, it could be that the situation is actually the opposite for a short while. It could be that Jakob challenges Karla in the way he varies his musical initiatives. In relation to the description of what is happening at around no. 7 in the scores, for example, the video recording reveals that Jakob plays with a flat hand and that he leaves his hand on the djembe for a short while after each beat. The feeling is that by doing so, Jakob makes a statement challenging Karla to follow up on his playing. (The video recording visualizes the fact that Karla follows up by hitting the djembe with a light, "jumping" hand.) He shows, in other words, that he can express himself distinctly and in a personal way through the music.

The fascinating aspect is that, presuming that Jakob can make this variation consciously, he must be aware that turn-taking is going on and that he is able to influence it creatively. In this way, the music therapy improvisation becomes a way for him to chart his own interaction possibilities.

There is, however, a constant struggle toward synchronization between musical and bodily actions between the two of them. This is indicated, for instance, in the scores where the dotted lines indicate in which direction the musical initiatives are regulated, that is, whether it is Karla who imitates Jakob or vice versa.

> Karla gets the feeling that they are both apart and together at the same time. Is it Jakob who plays randomly with her, next to her, for him, for her? Does he feel that she plays with him, next to him, for herself, for him?

After this section, it seems that Karla tries to prolong Jakob's level of conscious turn-taking by incorporating his playing into a longer musical phrase as she actively accompanies his actions (see nos. 9–13 in the scores). However, he gets tired and is no longer able to maintain the same amount of concentration (something which seems evident as he gets unsettled at around no. 10 in the scores).

> Karla feels that they are having a "real" discussion: Jakob has his arguments and she has hers, yet the discussion is without a transparent conclusion. Karla sees that Jakob gets tired; he sweats and struggles to keep his body in an upright position, and she feels that her energy also runs out. She tries to find a suitable moment to end their playing, one not too untimely for Jakob, which again reminds her of how difficult it is to end a session with him; her trying to make a musical statement and him—despite his tiredness—always wanting more ...

> (Here Karla painted two fingers pointing at each other, as in Michelangelo's painting Creation of Adam.)

The way Karla varies her rhythmical playing can be interpreted as (1) variations of her inviting Jakob into the playing, or (2) varied attempts to adjust her music to Jakob's expressions. Probably it is both, and hence Karla uses the rhythmical aspect to both observe and adjust herself to Jakob and at the same time try out possible areas of interaction.

The large degree to which pauses are used, including the amount of time that Jakob and Karla use to listen to each other in this excerpt, reflects that there is a sensitive adaptation process going on between them. This reveals that they are both trying to find out something about the other and that they are trying to establish a space for interaction.

BOTH EXCERPTS

In both excerpts, Jakob moves his arms a lot. It is probable that Jakob's unconscious arm movements over time become conscious, for example, as a conscious way of taking the initiative and making a response. In this sense, the music therapy improvisation balances on Jakob's zone of proximal development, continuously challenging him to develop and master more.

In general, interaction and turn-taking are a major aspect in both excerpts of the improvisation. To characterize this aspect, concepts such as dialogue ("powerful dialogue," "intense dialogue"), conversation, communication ("amazing communication"), and synchronization are used in the descriptions. (Rhythm is suggested to create the main dynamic force of change.)

As dialogue, the improvisation is described as alternating between musical and/or relational in that Karla and Jakob are "intertwined and at their most playful and are at a more expressive and meaningful way of being" and hence is imprinted with joy, happiness, desire, and strong feelings from both of them through "attuned rhythmic playing and vocalization" and "sensitive and unburdening playing."

Although it is noticed that it is Karla who mainly "waits," invites, and gives Jakob "space for response," it is not always clear whether it is Karla or Jakob who takes the initiative and gives the response in the turn-taking, or who imitates whom.

Two concepts are drafted throughout the observations of the two excerpts: One is "space" and the other is "silence"/"pause." The creating of "spaces" is something that several of the observers mention (in terms of both music and relation), and, most likely, "space" refers to the music therapy improvisation affording meaningful interaction.

This implies that Jakob and Karla receive each other's expressions, whether musically, bodily, or emotionally or by sympathizing and empathizing. This is, for instance, very directly expressed from one observer as he/she puts him-/herself in Jakob's place in order "to feel what he feels" and to "join him in his challenges."

Also, another observer suggests "projective identification." Karla is also described as "direct, reflecting some of the bodily affect" in Jakob. Silence is mainly used in connection to action and intentions, such as before/after initiatives and responses, as an "alternating between tension and silences."

Jakob is described as enjoying the music and this way of being together. It is agreed that music has an impact on his body language and that he wants to resonate with the music. It is also agreed that he gives of himself but takes care of himself as well, that he seems to have an intuitive sense of phrasing, and that he expresses himself excitedly and spontaneously, mainly through body movements and gestures (which is sometimes described in detail by the observers).

Most of the observers have noticed that Jakob occasionally characteristically crosses his arms in front of his chest, and several of them have suggested what this might mean. One says that it is a way for him to "hold" himself (this is meant both directly and indirectly); another says that it is as if he reflects and responds at the same time.

Other movements are interpreted differently, and his finger-tapping and scratching on the drum skin are connected to a need to explore and described as an "interesting tactile response."

In addition, observers of Jakob's facial expression and body movements question whether Karla sometimes challenges him too much, such that he gets scared and ambivalent, for instance, when he moves his arms and grits his teeth.

Obviously, and according to all the observers, his readiness is evident in the way he moves, shows tensions, and uses his voice, all of which are aspects that Karla activates and mirrors in her music.

As for Karla, she is characterized as "sympathetic and confident" and one who supports and observes Jakob as a whole but also sees him in detail. It is noticed that she reflects and makes Jakob feel safe, while simultaneously opening up for him to interact. (One observer sees that she smiles as she imitates Jakob's movements.)

Karla uses her whole body to communicate, by moving her arms and hands a lot and by leaning back to indicate a finale. She also makes facial gestures with her vocalizing.

Karla's voice is understood as a salient aspect in her approach, in that it is "warm and flexible and picks up on Jakob's apparently 'noncontrolling movements' in her matching and changing."

Additionally, it is pointed out that Karla shows enthusiasm to meet Jakob, that she catches his attention and challenges him to communicate.

Yet sometimes Karla is described as taking a rather dominant role, that is, she challenges a great deal and is almost confrontational in her music, as if she "teases" Jakob to make him respond and "answer." In this sense, she seems to be too active sometimes and thereby causes overstimulation.

She is also criticized for being too "accomplished" in her use of the djembe. Several observers have noticed her use of professional techniques, for instance, the way she changes to reacting to and answering Jakob's actions, something that is recognized as being mother–infant-like.

The way Karla waits and listens before starting to play is commented upon as being effective to extend and develop the music therapy improvisation further while never leaving Jakob alone.

It is agreed that the turn-taking increases throughout the video recording, starting out as attuning in The Guitar Excerpt and maximized as a "finely tuned" reciprocal communication in The Djembe Excerpt, where Jakob and Karla play together in the same beat.

The Djembe Excerpt—in which both of them play on the same instrument and the physical distance between them is therefore very small—is imprinted with intimacy. In this excerpt, the nonverbal (also expressed as "preverbal" by the observers) attention and communication builds up affect in both of them as they develop the musical dialogue and interaction by playing and listening closely to each other.

Although it is sensed that Karla is working with Jakob on both conscious and unconscious levels, the process is typically described as a type of "musicalization" (my word) of responses in which aspects of rhythm, tonality, dynamics, meter, speed, form, and different register, as well as "chords juxtaposed with vocalizing," drive the music therapy improvisation onward.

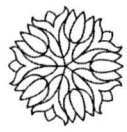

Chapter 5

SUMMING UP THE NARRATIVE

Perhaps not so surprisingly, it is turn-taking, dialogue, interaction, and communication which are the all-encompassing topics in the narrative, yet these are most often portrayed as a "musicalized" interaction or taking turns/dialogue/ communication.

This is a theme that is mainly recognized in the descriptions by the use of action words such as "attune," "adjust," "create space," "leave space," "challenge," "respond," "taking initiative," "withdraw," "coming forth," "build tension," "decrease intensity," "imitate," "synchronize," "mirror," "continue," "stop," "delay," "syncopate," "time (perfectly)," "juxtapose," "follow up," "move nearer," and "move away."

The perspective concerning time seemed to be prominent, too. As we can tell from the action words in the above paragraph, many of them are closely linked to time (e.g., "synchronize," "continue," "stop," "delay," "syncopate," "time," and "juxtapose"). I have grouped these descriptive aspects as "actions of musical-relational synchronizing."

Another related aspect connects to the way in which the musical-relational synchronizing was experienced as being interfered with by joy, challenge, ambivalence, and vitality, as if it were actually "magnetic" for the observers. Mostly the topic is characterized pleasantly, either as playful, meaningful, or expressive, but also it is questioned for being sometimes "too" stimulating, "too" challenging and confronting.

Additionally, the breaks, which are mainly identified as "spaces" (pauses and silences were also used), are crucial in that they are experienced as "loaded," meaning by this that they are important and mean something in the turn-taking.

The personal imprint is evidential, in that the observers (including me) use "I feel" and "I sense" in the descriptions.

Something that frames the next aspect is that the observers in a fundamental way confront the improvisation as a way to explore interaction itself. Paradoxically, then, the interaction turned out to be entwined in the music therapy improvisation as a point of departure, means, and goal.

Another interesting aspect is the seemingly direct link between action and intention in the narrative. This could stem from a willingness in the observers to interpret the client's bodily actions as intentional (e.g., that his arm movements mean something), as well as the opposite, that the client's intentions come out musically (e.g., that he "tells his story" through the music).

Still, rather than to conclude or appoint an action's intention, there is a tendency among the observers to make reservations or to hold open several/other interpretations, something that is explained by the extended use of verbs such as "expect" and "assume" in the descriptions. In fact, several times, the descriptions are articulated as questions, through which the observers leave the interpretations "up in the air."

As a result, action and interaction are seen as a point of rotation for the music therapy improvisation. This may not be very surprising for many experienced music therapists.

A question emerges from the narrative: Is there a direct link between action and intention in the music therapy improvisation? The realization of this question could suggest that there really is a need to understand action as a phenomenon—in particular, the action–intention relationship—*before* predicting what music therapy improvisation can lead to in terms of a therapeutic outcome.

The last aspect concerns the apparent confusion in the observations connected to the question regarding who takes the initiative and who gives the response in the interaction. Normally, I have thought of this as typical for any musical interplay, where the musicians through the music meld together as one expression. In a music therapy perspective, however, the disturbing part is realizing that the disagreement reveals a problem connected to a good reconstruction of all of the aspects in the interaction process since, obviously, it is sometimes important to know whether a client really takes the initiative or not.

At the same time, it also reveals the degree of complexity connected to interaction as a phenomenon, which in turn teaches me that there are particular aspects regarding interaction as a phenomenon that also deserve a closer elaboration. I question whether a discussion about this belongs at theoretical levels that are closer to philosophy.

The interaction aspects need to be treated generally, yet without losing the genuine sound of music therapy improvisation as a phenomenon, because, after all, the type of interaction that I was dealing with was musical, not verbal.

Eventually, it seems that music therapy improvisation, as is true with any human interaction, is imprinted with an existential quality. Could Bakhtin help me to abstract this aspect theoretically and philosophically?

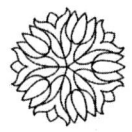

Chapter 6

INTRODUCING MIKHAIL BAKHTIN AND HIS CONTEXT

ABOUT BAKHTIN

Russian linguist and language researcher Mikhail Mikhailovich Bakhtin (1895–1975) was one of the leading thinkers of the 20th century, according to Holquist (1990), the Bakhtin scholar. Bakhtin's ideas can be seen as a result of the worldwide movement of alternative philosophy and pedagogy that was going on after the Russian Revolution (White & Peters, 2011). It is especially his notion of dialogue that has influenced the thinking of many people from various fields—not just from linguistics, but also from philosophy, sociology, pedagogy, the arts, and so forth.

The Basis of Dialogue

I have learned that Bakhtin developed many of his ideas on dialogue in the 1920s and 1930s, in the aftermath of the Russian Revolution. Slaatelid (1998) refers to Tzvetan Todorov and his book *Mikhail Bakhtine: Le principe dialogique,* wherein it is suggested that Bakhtin (and his dialogue) went through five periods of development from around 1920 to the last part of the 1970s.

The first periods consisted of a phenomenological period and a sociological period. After that came the linguistic period and a period in which literature history was emphasized. In the fifth and last period, all four previous periods emerged into one synthesis. One of his last projects, which he never finished, was to write a methodology for the human sciences (cf. Slaatelid, 1998).

Lately, thinkers within art and therapy, especially those who place their ideas within the perspectives of cultural psychology and cultural sociology, have also started to refer to Bakhtin. It is his perspectives on human existence and expression, and in particular his communicative ethics and the position of the Self, that they discuss (see, e.g., Leiman, 2011).

Reading Bakhtin

Reading Bakhtin is challenging. When explaining dialogue and other central concepts, Bakhtin uses complex meta-language. Not even Bakhtin scholars always agree on how to understand him. In her keynote in the Bakhtin 2014 conference in Stockholm, one of the most prominent Bakhtin scholars, Caryl Emerson, discussed the complexity of Bakhtin's ideas. She said that his ideas always seemed to resist a final definition and that Bakhtin probably *opposed* formalization of his thinking. This could explain why Bakhtin never labeled his reflections with terms such as "theory" or "philosophy."

I find reading Bakhtin to be both difficult and very inspiring at the same time. Descriptions by Jayne White and Michael Peters (2011), editors of *Bakhtinian Pedagogy: Opportunities and Challenges for Research, Policy, and Practice in Education Across the Globe*, fit well with my experiences. They say (p. 1) that "reading Bakhtin is a literary experience that leaves the reader gasping for air yet wanting more" and that his ideas are "elusive, foreign, and dark, while at the same time alluring, hopeful, and joyous." Therefore, for Bakhtin lovers who are not members of his circle, to read him "call[s] us to a place of instability and confusion," and for those who attempt to interpret his ideas in a practical sense, as I do in this book, there is "unnerving appeal and challenge"—a mood with "multicultural allusions and subtexts."

It also should be said that Bakhtin himself could have been afraid of being misread. After all, he experienced that the Russian State Accrediting Bureau first denied his doctoral thesis with the title *Rabelais and the Folk Culture of the Middle Ages and Renaissance*, which was an interpretation of French renaissance writer Rabelais and his philosophy. Because they read his concept of dialogue as a criticism of Stalin and his monologue's power and governance, Bakhtin was put into exile for many years. He therefore wrote under pseudonyms for a long time.

However, Bakhtin had many friends and academic groups who were influenced by his ideas and helped him toward an acceptance of the doctoral work. Eventually, Bakhtin's doctoral work was approved and published in 1965, 19 years after its first rejection.

Who and What Inspired Bakhtin?

Bakhtin's ideas were situated; they belong to a time and place and must therefore be read as products of the sphere that gave life to them. White and Peters (2011) understand Bakhtin's dialogical ideas in relation to his attention to the Russian philosophy of life through which language draws from multiple meanings and ideologies in play.

Brandist (2011) finds a line from the dialogue of Socrates/Plato to neo-Kantian philosophers like Apel and Habermas, to Heidegger, Gadamer, Hegel, Freire, Kierkegaard, Buber, and Wittgenstein, to Bakhtin (and Voloshinov).

Bakhtin developed his dialogue long before Freire presented his classic *Pedagogy of the Oppressed* in the 1960s, but like Freire's agenda, Bakhtin's was also political. Equality of speech was the idea; he aimed to teach the masses to speak publicly, to create a population that could engage actively in a new democratic society (Brandist, 2011).

White and Peters (2011) believe that Bakhtin's attention to morality is an outcry of his Kantian and religious background, coupled with his experiences in Stalinist Russia (remember that Bakhtin was in exile). This could explain how Bakhtin calls the reader to reflect on his treatment of Other as a responsive and accountable act of the self. They think that through such interaction, Bakhtin urges his readers to consider their relational impact on Other and their potential to give and receive from such encounter.

In this regard, "Bakhtinian interpretations are responsible acts that are highly reflexive in nature. They are eternally answerable, since they are always in process of becoming" (White & Peters, 2011, pp. 6–7). Such a stance, they say, can be deeply confronting and alarmingly frustrating in the contemporary era of certainty that characterizes much of Western ideology. White and Peters (2011) suggest that instead of becoming perplexed by all this, we can be provoked into action and to applying Bakhtin's ideas to aspects of contemporary experiences.

The Bakhtin Circles

Today, there are several so-called Bakhtin circles around the world in which communities of intellectual scholars (from linguistics, mostly) come together to discuss and elaborate upon Bakhtin's ideas.

Interestingly, Craig Brandist (2011), the well-known Bakhtin scholar, says that the first Bakhtin circle started as a Kantian seminar in

Germany before it moved to the Belorussian town of Vitebsk, where Bakhtin gathered with many radical artists. Under their influence, the circle became an arena into which the participants brought ideas from the various projects in which they were engaged and reflected on them in a dialogical fashion (Slaatelid, 1998).

Typically, Bakhtin thus developed his ideas along with fruitful opposition from other scholars from many fields. The Bakhtin circle became a discussion circle with many radical artists and scholars, not least of whom was literary scholar Pavel Medvedev, who was organizing an Institute of Arts and Humanities and Institute of the Living Word in Petrograd/Leningrad.

From the beginning, the members of the Bakhtin circle played formative roles, and many of them, like Bakhtin, combined research and teaching. They understood education as something embedded in general social processes and cultural activities and cultural activities; pedagogy became *social pedagogy* (Brandist, 2011, xi). This pedagogy has a long history of holistic education that educated "head, heart, and hands" as a harmonious unity, which was influenced by Swiss educator Johann H. Pestalozzi (1756–1827).

Lived Experiences?

As a curiosity, École d'Humanité, the Swiss boarding school that I attended in 1978–1979, was an example of the more radical type of such a socially and humanistically oriented pedagogy. I realize now that I might actually have lived experiences of attending a dialogically centered school environment, and of a pedagogy system that encouraged student discussion and collaboration and placed heavy emphasis on the arts. I am sure my attraction to Bakhtin and his world has derived from these experiences.

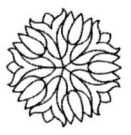

Chapter 7

CONCERNING MY TRANSPOSING OF INSIGHTS OF BAKHTIN'S IDEAS

MY PERSPECTIVE

Bakhtin's name has been mentioned in music therapy texts by Ansdell (2014), Ansdell and Pavlicevic (2005), Garred (2004), and Stige (2002), but as far as I know, my PhD thesis from 2008 includes the most extensive elaboration thus far.

Caryl Emerson and Michael Holquist, editors of *The Dialogic Imagination* (Bakhtin, 1981), the large collection of Bakhtin essays, underline that Bakhtin's ideas belong to a context and that his language therefore deserves a detailed study. This is not something any reader of his works can ignore. Where does this leave me and my use of Bakhtin's ideas?

Bringing Bakhtin's Ideas into Dialogue with Other Traditions

Brandist (2011) argues that Bakhtin's ideas transcend the limitations of his politics. In contrast to other Bakhtin scholars (e.g., Slaatelid, 1998) who claim that there is a reductionist recirculation of Bakhtin's terminology going on, Brandist (2011) says that Bakhtin's ideas do not have to be seen only in relation to their history. It is also a good idea to bring Bakhtinian ideas into dialogue with other traditions and welcome reflection on current educational practices from an appropriate critical distance.

Reading Brandist (2011) empowered me in the process of the present book. For me, working as a music therapist and reflecting upon it through my research and with the lenses of Bakhtin's philosophy are answerable acts; they have a social agenda and are in a continuous process of becoming.

However, I am aware that my elaboration involves risks of reduction and simplification. It is a weakness in my elaboration that Bakhtin's ideas were meant for language and people's use of language and not a type of communication that is developed through musical improvisation. It might therefore be helpful to redefine "language" to include music, body language, and gestures when reading this book.

Communicative Being and Communicative Repairing

Bakhtin himself emphasizes that dialogue involves us all totally, with our body and mind in time and place. According to his philosophy, communication almost *is* existence and vice versa. Bakhtin and I share the view that communication in all forms is vital to existence; communication describes us as human beings.

However, as a music therapist, I have seen how fragile communication is. When communication fails, we fail as human beings, too. For some people and/or in some phases of life, people's abilities and/or possibilities to communicate are poor. In these cases, the communication needs support. Sometimes it needs mending, too.

Music therapy theorists occasionally define music therapy as a type of *communication repairing* (e.g., Ansdell, 2014). I like to think that Bakhtin would have been interested in my creative use of his ideas for the benefit of optimizing people's health and involvement with others and the world.

I argue that many aspects of his dialogical world deserve to be transposed to music therapy, and in particular to improvisation. His philosophy not only shows us the nature of human existence, but also calls on us to act aesthetically and ethically with our whole self. By being responsive toward ourselves and others, we must ask questions, heed, respond, agree, and so forth, even in situations when communication is difficult:

> In this dialogue, a person participates wholly and throughout his whole life: with his eyes, lips, hands, soul, spirit, with his whole body and deeds (Bakhtin, 1984, p. 293).

Interestingly, Jostein Børtnes (2001), the Norwegian Bakhtin scholar, says that Bakhtin's dialogue relates to the word *protivopolozjnost* in Russian, which in an etymological sense means "dialogical opposition/resistance" (p. 97). This, says Børtnes, involves being directed toward each other, not necessarily (just) as opponents, but face-to-face, and thus it includes body expressions, gestures, and mimicry. This image of dialogue is meaningful in a music therapy context like the one for this book, not just when the client in the narrative is without words and therefore is more dependent on the body language, but also because the music therapist tends to "read" a client's body movements as part of his/her overall language.

As music therapists, we would perhaps say that gestures and body expressions sometimes constitute some clients' "first language." For a client like Jakob, who has severe multiple handicaps, this is evident: His body language is a natural and intuitive way of unfolding, expressing himself, and responding and hence framing his "word repertoire."

United in a Pragmatically Oriented Science Philosophy

I must reiterate that Bakhtin was referring to texts. I transfer his ideas to people and music, which are not reducible to his voices–ideas, as in novels. As Matusov (2015) states, in novels, authors can legitimately injure or even kill their characters. This is, of course, unthinkable in music therapy, which involves real-life events with real people who need support and help.

Also, we must remember that Bakhtin's dialogical universe is a worldview, and one might again ask if, when, and how his ideas are transferable to micro-settings and responsiveness in music therapy improvisation. I find it fruitful to sympathize with Holquist (1990), who suggests interpretations of Bakhtin's theories to be a *pragmatically oriented science philosophy*. It is "one of several modern epistemologies that seek to grasp human behavior through the use humans make of language" (p. 15), or communication, as I would put it. Bakhtin's "real" project then unifies with mine in the degree to which it aims to understand human actions and behavior in communication.

My transposing of insights of his ideas to music therapy will sometimes be closer to his ideas, sometimes further away, but as long as I am transparent about my positioning, my project is fair.

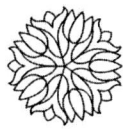

Chapter 8

MIKHAIL BAKHTIN'S TERMINOLOGY

I will now present the terms in Bakhtin's philosophy that I find most valuable to music therapy in general and to improvisation in particular. I introduce the terms "answerability" and "dialogue" first. These are the key concepts that in turn influence Bakhtin's terms such as "action," "relation," "the Other," "utterance," "authorship," "polyphony," "voice," and "ventriloquism." At the end, I will present another core term of his, "carnival," which is closely connected to his notion of "laughter."

ANSWERABILITY

In his short essay *Art and Answerability*, Bakhtin (1990) articulated the importance of answerability. Bakhtin says in this essay that there are three domains of human culture. These are: (1) science or reason, (2) ethics or the life of action, and (3) art or aesthetics (Bakhtin, 1990). These three can be united in an individual, but this unity can be either external or internal.

"Answerability" is Bakhtin's term for the process of mutual response, answering, that happens between two persons or between art and life. An inner connection between art and life affords answerability, in the meaning of responsiveness to others, events, and the world. Through a process of consistent response, or answerability, art and life can be unified by and in the person.

The need to answer the other responsibly implies obligation, and such obligation involves an individual's concrete response to actual persons in specific situations. Thus, for Bakhtin, "answerability" is the name for individual responsibility and obligation that leads to action for ourselves and also on behalf of others.

Answerability, Juxwik (2004) elaborates, highlights the unique responsibility that characterizes the individual's responses to others in everyday interaction and in textual production. My idea, which will be presented and discussed in the chapter 10, is that answerability is reflected on some levels in the music therapy improvisation with Jakob and Karla, too.

Answerability and Addressivity

Bakhtin scholars such as Holquist (1990) and Slaatelid (1998) think that Bakhtin's "addressivity" in large part unifies with "answerability," which covers the idea of Bakhtin's existential project. Holquist (1990) says that Bakhtin would describe this as follows:

> We are alive and human to the degree that we are answerable, i.e., to the degree that we can respond to addressivity. We cannot choose not to be in dialogue, not only with other human beings, but also with the natural and cultural figurations we lump together as "the world." (p. 29)

Matusov (2015, p. 401) has coined the concept of "interaddressivity" to capture people's inherent ontological interest in each other. This refers to a constant expectation of being surprised by the other, by his/her strangeness. He thinks that for Bakhtin, the opaqueness of human consciousnesses has ethical primacy over the principle of the transparency of/among consciousnesses, because it promotes interest in and respect for the Other.

The idea is, "If I can never fully know the consciousness of another person at any given moment for any given issue, I should treasure and be interested in the other person" (Matusov, 2015, p. 399). This implies that ...

> *I* need *the Other* only until *I* have fully understood *Him or Her*. As soon as *my* consciousness can consume the consciousness of *the Other* either via the meaning content and/or via the meaning generation process, *I* do not need *the Other*. Our consciousnesses converge at least partially. The more *I* become knowledgeable, the more *I* become independent of *the Other*, and the more *the Other* becomes redundant and unnecessary for *me*. *The understood Other* is redundant and, thus, can be eliminated. Perceived-to-be-fully-understood

people are dispensable and replicable. (Matusov, 2015, p. 399, author's italics)

As Bakhtin repeated many times in his essays and books, the sense of the interconnectedness of self and other, text and context, art and daily life forms the foundation of the creative process and what creates the center of answerability.

Answerability as Active Engagement

Answerability requires active engagement with one's situation. In fact, answerability is where the uniqueness of each individual originates. Answerability invokes the need of dialogues between selves who act to answer others' actions. In answering the world around them, selves imbue their responses with unrepeatable intonations to impart new meanings. The distinctiveness and creativity of each response underlie the act of life authoring as answerability. What defines an act is the degree and kind of personal responsibility that one assumes for it (Morson & Emerson, 1990). Clark and Holquist (1984, p. 9, my italics) summarize: "What the self is answerable *to* is the social environment; what the self is answerable *for* is the authorship of its responses."

DIALOGUE

"Dialogue" is a term that followed and took over for "answerability." I will refer to dialogue in the following pages before returning to answerability again in chapter 15.

Bakhtin never finally defined "dialogue." Dialogue is a concept he developed and changed throughout his lifetime. This leads to several possible ways to approach it.

Linguistically, the word "dialogue" is composed of the prefix *dia-*, which means "through," and the suffix *-logue*, which derives from the Greek "logos," meaning "words." This indicates that "dialogue" originally connected to communication through words, which could explain why Bakhtin, as a linguist, chooses the term.

Dialogue Inspiration

Yet, and as we have learned already, dialogue was also a large concept of his time, both in philosophy (especially in the German Marburger school and through Kant and his philosophy) and politics (Marx, among others). It is well known that these thinkers influenced Bakhtin. Ansdell and Pavlicevic (2005) suggest that a roll call of such (dialogue) philosophers who could inspire music therapy would include "Hegel, Novalis, Freud, Dilthey, Husserl, Jaspers, Heidegger, Merleau-Ponty, Levinas, Buber, Gadamer, Wittgenstein, Adorno, Bakhtin, Bohm, Kristeva—taking us from German idealism to contemporary constructionism" (p. 204).

Influences from Buber's Dialogue

Bakhtin (2003) admits that he is influenced by Socrates but says that he owes Martin Buber and other former dialogue philosophers his gratitude. There are striking similarities between Bakhtin's "dialogue" and Buber's "dialogue," particularly in the way in which Buber presents the term in his book *I and Thou* (Buber, 1992). Buber's philosophy is a point of departure in Rudy Garred's (2006) work in music therapy. The largest difference between Bakhtin and Buber (and in many ways, Levinas, too, as we shall soon see later on in chapter 9) is that to Buber, dialogue is not possible without imagining God, whereas to Bakhtin, who was also a religious man, dialogue exists primarily between people and because of people. Bakhtin's "dialogue" therefore requires embodiment through live situations.

In contrast to Buber, Bakhtin draws a larger attention toward external events and toward what people do; in other words, his interest lies in human action and interaction, not merely in the internal processes. "Truth," Bakhtin states, "is not to be found inside the head of an individual person; it is born between people collectively searching for the truth in the process of their dialogic interaction" (Bakhtin, in Shotter, 1999, p. 184) and with the person's entire and active participation in the world with others (Bakhtin, 1984).

Dialogue as Existence

"Existence," for Bakhtin, becomes the event of co-being, which manifests itself in the form of a constant, ceaseless creation and exchange of meaning. "Being," for Bakhtin, is the simultaneity of a co-being. In other words, dialogue becomes an endless existential social project.

Bakhtin in this way adds another tone to the term, which is innovative and vitalizing: "Dialogue" is simply a way to define a human being's relation to another human being. Hence a human being uses language not merely as a means of expression, but also to communicate and to be in dialogue (Bakhtin, 1986b). In this sense, dialogue is not just the basis for existence; it is also its goal and purpose.

In the following presentation of other Bakhtinian concepts, we must remember that this notion of dialogue is the lodestar.

OTHER RELATED CONCEPTS

Bakhtin's Action

In his dialogue, Bakhtin emphasizes "action," meaning action between people who direct their attention toward each other. Thus, in dialogue, action insists on a co-action in joint attention. Just as an utterance is directed toward someone, action in dialogue refers to being actively engaged, face-to-face, in a live situation.

Claiming that we cannot relate to what is within each individual, Bakhtin (1998) says that action is what we have and what we can relate to. Addressing another person is addressing through action while being involved in a personal sense.

In other words, an action demands personal commitment, or embodiment, as he would call it (Bakhtin, 1986a). This suggests that utterances exist only as embodied utterances between persons and their actions. Apparently, this explains why "everything" in Bakhtin's dialogue is a response/answer and how a response primarily requires action, not in the sense of problem-solving, but in the sense of relating. This relating includes relating to one's own self and one's own answerability (see "Answerability" above).

Relation

What gives Bakhtin's dialogue such a central position is precisely the kind of relation that conversations manifest: the conditions that must be met if any exchange between different speakers is to occur at all. Since Bakhtin did not define the term "relation" himself, Holquist (1990) suggests his understanding of relation to cover its definition:

> Relation is most economically defined as one in which differences—while still remaining different—serve as the building blocks of simultaneity. [...] It is this mutuality of

differences that makes dialogue Bakhtin's master concept, for it is present in exchanges at all levels—between words in language, people in society, organisms in ecosystems, and even between processes in the natural world. (p. 40)

I understand that it is the personal differences merging into mutuality through dialogue that Bakhtin accentuates here. This process is complex and demands fine-tuning, and relation is the basis around which dialogue arises. [Trondalen (2016) describes in her book *Relational music therapy: An intersubjective perspective* how the fine-tuning could be applied in music therapy.]

The Other

Today, the Self and the organization of Self receive much attention within newer psychological and sociological theory. This is also the case in music therapy, with its import of theories from developmental psychology, especially Stern (see, e.g., Trondalen, 2016).

It would be going beyond the scope of this book to go into the details of a presentation of theories of the Self. The essential part here is that to Bakhtin, dialogue enacts a drama containing more than one actor. Therefore, Self is above all dialogical, a relation that is not static but is about to be (or about to end).

Bakhtin almost changes the picture by moving the role of the Other to the forefront. This is visible, for instance, in the following citation:

To be means to be for another, and through the other, for oneself. A person has no internal sovereign territory, he is wholly and always on the boundary; looking inside himself, he looks into the eyes of another with the eyes of another. (Bakhtin, 1984, p. 287)

As we can see, the image of an addressee is crucial. In fact, everything a person does is understood in relation to an addressee. No utterance, no voice, not even an action is possible without an addressee. This begins with the fact that a word is half someone else's. It becomes "one's own" only when the speaker populates it with his own intention, his own accent, when he appropriates the word, adapting it to his own semantic and expressive intention (Bakhtin, 1981, pp. 293–294).

In Bakhtin's imagination, there are several possible Others, since dialogue is seen as external (between two people) or internal (between an earlier and a later self). Who makes the utterance in the dialogue, however, remains unclear. Bakhtin puts the question this way: Whose voice is being heard? (Bakhtin, 1981). He suggests that although the voice belongs to "you," it is not sure that "you" own the meaning. Instead, there is (always) a complex interaction of voices and meaning.

Bakhtin's Architectonic Model of the Human Psyche

To better understand the complexity connected to the various dialogical relations that Bakhtin outlines, it is perhaps useful to mention his architectonic model of the human psyche (Bakhtin, 1993). This model has three components: "I-for-myself," "I-for-the-Other," and "Other-for-me." The first, the I-for-myself as a source of identity, is unreliable, says Bakhtin (1993). In fact, it is the I-for-the-Other through which human beings develop a sense of identity. This I-for-the-Other serves as an amalgamation of the way in which others view me (Bakhtin, 1993). Conversely, the Other-for-me describes the way in which others incorporate my perceptions of them into their own identities. Identity, as Bakhtin describes it here, does not belong merely to the individual; rather, it is shared by all.

The Utterance

Another essential concept in Bakhtin's dialogue is "utterance." Bakhtin says that an utterance is a unit of speech communication that cannot be invoked in general. A fundamental difference between Saussure, the French linguist, and Bakhtin regarding language is that Bakhtin understands "parole" as a social phenomenon while Saussure defines "parole" as the individual part.

According to Bakhtin (1986b), all utterances are social phenomena that express dialogical relations between persons. An utterance is of someone, for someone, and about someone and is ineluctably tied to someone within a situation (Bakhtin, 1986b).

In real-life dialogue, which is the simplest and the most classic form of speech communication, the change of speaking subjects (speakers) that determines the boundaries of the utterance is especially clear.

However, the same process occurs in other spheres of communication as well. Interestingly, Bakhtin adds that the nature of the boundaries of the utterance remains the same, even when including areas of "complexly organized cultural communication (scientific and artistic)" (Bakhtin, 1986b, p. 75). Bakhtin questions whether science manages to deal with utterances that are unrepeatable and unique and thus may resist generalization.

In trans-linguistics, a concept constructed by Bakhtin, the aim is to study the structures and the laws by which the utterances function, not their uniqueness. Each separate utterance is individual, of course, but each sphere in which language is used develops its own relatively stable types of utterances, or what Bakhtin calls "speech genres" (1986b, p. 60).

Bakhtin emphasizes that an utterance is demarked by the utterances that precede and follow it. It can range from a one-word exclamation or a nonverbal gesture to a complete novel (1986b, p. 60). To conclude, utterances form the stuff of a living and developing discourse between embodied, socially organized persons.

Heteroglossia

"Heteroglossia" is one of Bakhtin's key terms. It describes the coexistence of distinct varieties within a single "language" (in Greek: *hetero-,* meaning "different," and *glōssa,* meaning "tongue, language"); in this way, the term translates the Russian разноречие ("raznorechie"; literally, "different-speech-ness").[12]

Bakhtin viewed the modern novel as a literary form best suited for the exploitation of heteroglossia (1986b, p. 60). He gives an example of an illiterate peasant, who speaks church Slavonic to God, speaks to his family in their own peculiar dialect, sings songs in yet a third (!), and attempts to emulate officious high-class dialect when he dictates petitions to the local government.

Bakhtin identifies a specific type of discourse, the "authoritative discourse," which demands to be assimilated by the reader or listener. Examples might be religious dogma, scientific theory, or a popular book. He views this type of discourse as past, finished, and hierarchically superior, and therefore demands "unconditional allegiance" rather than accepting interpretation (1986b, p. 60). However, authoritative discourse plays an insignificant role in the novel: Because it is not open to interpretation, it cannot enter into hybrid utterance (Bakhtin, 1981).

I will be careful with my use of the term "heteroglossia" in the present book. I understand it is an intricate term within the field of linguistics. A general impression is that heteroglossia suggests that everything has meaning, which in itself means that everything is understood to be part of a greater (and complex) whole.

On a micro level, the music therapy improvisation between Jakob and Karla could be seen as a dialect of a specific type of speech. As a musician, when I perform songs to the accompaniment of my own guitar-playing, I play differently than when I play as a music therapist. Both situations require different "speech-nesses" or, rather, "music-nesses" (my word), when different types of voices would be present in me.

Voices and Polyphony

Two well-known notions in Bakhtin's philosophy are voices and polyphony. In some ways, they are related.

The way in which Bakhtin uses the first term, "voices," is complex. For him, voices are understood more generally as discourses, ideologies, perspectives, or themes, and as meaning-making (Baxter, 2011). Voices, then, are something much more than a solo musical voice or a tune; instead, they are the interplay of those voices, where opposition and dissonances also occur.

Bakhtin defines "polyphony" by referring to the value of open-ended and polysemic texts. Although he initially borrowed the term from music theory, it was his readings and interpretations of the novels of Dostoevsky that enabled him to develop it. Bakhtin's thesis is that the affirmation of someone else's consciousness is a core aspect in Dostoevsky's work. He notes that all voices are important and that the structure is open-ended and polyphonic.

As human beings, we are in his picture constantly in an unfinalized process of individuals' voices where there is no last word:

> There is neither a first nor a last word, and there are no limits to the dialogic context (it extends into the boundless past and boundless future). Even *past* meanings, that is, those born in the dialogue of past centuries, can never be stable (finalized, ended once and for all)—they will always change (be renewed) in the process of subsequent, future development of the dialogue. At any moment in the development of the dialogue, there are immense, boundless masses of forgotten contextual meanings, but at certain moments of the dialogue's subsequent development along the way, they are recalled and invigorated in renewed form (in a new context). (Bakhtin, 1986b, p. 170)

It is the unfinalization of the individual voices that creates true polyphony. Truth (which Bakhtin refers to as polyphonic truth and/or true dialogue) is not a statement, a phrase, or a musical chorus played by any of them. A single mouth cannot express it, just as a single mind cannot express it. The voices carry (only) partial truths that can complement each other. A number of different voices do not, however, make the truth simply if synthesized. It is their addressivity, engagement, and commitment to the context of a real-life event that distinguishes truth from untruth. The latter underlines the need for personal commitment and engagement in the situation.

Bakhtin points out, however, that voices and the negotiation of meanings are intimately intersected with the situation in which they are performed. A voice therefore has meaning *within* a context, but only together with other voices. Thus, the voice of "I" can mean what "I" say (or vocalize or play, for that matter), but only indirectly, since it is never solely responsible for its utterance and the meaning implied.

Typically, there is a constant interaction of meanings: "Which will affect the other, how it will do so, and to what degree is what is actually settled at the moment of utterance" (Bakhtin, 1981, p. 426). All meanings involved therefore have the potential to condition others. In other words, dialogue can never escape its situation. This matter also relates to another key term of Bakhtin's, "chronotope," which in short deals with time and place (Bakhtin, 1981).

Ventriloquism

To give an idea of the complexity of dialogue, Bakhtin introduces the process of ventriloquism. In a view grounded in ventriloquism, the very act of speaking precludes any claims about the individual being independent of society. According to Wetherell (2001), the linguist and Bakhtin scholar, interference and subordination are especially evident in the process of ventriloquism. It reflects the sociocultural situation of those doing the understanding. Hence ventriloquism gives a picture of the difficulties of being able to tell who actually speaks, whose voice is being spoken, and whose meanings are owned in the sound of the voices. The doll, to which the ventriloquist gives life through his own voice, confuses matters. Again, whose voice is being heard? Whose meaning does the doll's voice represent? Although the voice belongs to the ventriloquist, it sounds as if it comes from the doll and therefore functions as a realization of somebody else's voice.

Authorship

For Bakhtin, there is always a dominant energy (which could be an individual) in the aesthetics, which he terms "author." The other energy belongs to "hero." There is always a fundamental asymmetry in the roles of author and hero. While hero is involved in worldviews and knowledge of ordinary life, author is the aesthetic form itself [cf. Kruse's (2016) description of the will of the art and artist in chapter 1].

Bakhtin (1986b) says that "the author is a uniquely active form-giving energy, present not as a consciousness psychologically conceived, but in a stably meaningful cultural product" (p. 12). Although he (Bakhtin, 1984) refers to Dostoevsky's novels and their intense struggle of ideas as polyphony and beautiful form, he also says that a human act is a potential text that could be understood as a creative and aesthetic act, that is, as a human act and not a physical action (Bakhtin, 1986a).

Bakhtin illustrates a series of dilemmas relating to what we consider "author" in relation to a work produced. These involve the historical conditions of production, criticism disputes, and translation policies (Pampa, 2014). Pampa (2014), in his reading on Bakhtin, explains that the question of author in the work is subject to numerous theoretical sieges: author as character, as ideologist of the architectonics, as masked voice, as polyphonic ear, and so on.

The meta-language that Bakhtin uses to explain author and hero in novels is very complex, but an essence of it, as I understand it and have alluded to before, is bringing art closer to life. This process is one in which the spirit of (aesthetic) form is important. The idea pervading this all is that the author only exists in the dialogical context of its time (as a rejoinder, as a semantic position, as a system of motives) (Pampa, 2014).

Authorship thus requires creativity and genuine interest in the work and happens as a unique and unrepeatable event in the life of a text. Bakhtin's ideas engage a formidable theoretical project for the study of the humanities in general and of everyday language and artistic language in particular, says Pampa (2014).

CARNIVAL

One term that I find very interesting for my understanding of music therapy improvisation is Bakhtin's "carnival." Along with "dialogue," "carnival" is a major term for Bakhtin and one that pervades his whole thinking.

Bakhtin suggests the idea that the symbols in carnival have been transferred to our time and still exist in literature (Bakhtin, 1981, 1986a, 2003). For Bakhtin, carnival refers to a literary mode that subverts and liberates the assumptions of the dominant style or atmosphere through humor, the grotesque, chaos, and/or joy. The term "carnivalesque" is tied to the body and the public exhibition of its more private function.

Bakhtin reintroduces the medieval carnival as the popular laughter culture. In the medieval carnival, which was completely free from religion and politics, people could realize feelings, dreams, and utopian ideas that were normally perceived as immoral, insensible, or irrational. Normality was repelled while the carnival existed, and people could actually live the life of which they dreamed, freely, uninhibitedly, and in contrast to the suppressed conditions they were used to. (Medieval times were governed by rigid laws and extreme morality.)

Carnival's Ability to Regenerate and Revitalize Life

It is especially the idea of this carnival's ability to regenerate and revitalize life that pervades this work, an aspect that is especially interesting for therapy. Carnival (and carnivalesque literature, as Bakhtin claims) creates threshold situations where regular conventions are broken or reversed and genuine dialogue becomes possible. This creates a world upside down, where ideas and truths are tested and contested and all demand equal dialogical status.

Carnival affects all people, attracting them to the behavior and the rituals typical in it (Bakhtin, 1986a). Everyone is an active participant and everyone communes in the carnival act. It is very serious and very joyful at the same time. Therefore, carnival represents a stage for unfolding and provides opportunities for action that are particularly uncommon and unprecedented.

Bakhtin (2003) also suggests that carnival is the context in which distinct individual voices are heard; it is where they flourish and interact. While in Dostoevsky, life is existential dialogue, in carnival, life is the triumph of a vitality of the lowest order, the life of the flesh. It is the play of the unincarnated spirits of bodily elements, "a play wholly unfettered by the artist's will" (Shepherd, 1998, p. 92).

Laughter

The basis of laughter gives rise to carnival rituals that are also recognizable in modern times. Real laughter, however, is universal and has an ambivalent character (Bakhtin, 2003). It characterizes the carnival through parody, irony, and what Bakhtin calls "grotesque realism," which implies degradation. This means that everything that is *up*, like the spiritual, idealistic, and abstract, is brought down to earth, to where bodies appear in an unbroken unit.

Laughter does not negate the serious, but purifies and replenishes it. It therefore attracts the public into the material bodily celebration of carnival. Bakhtin asserts that as a distanced image, a subject cannot be comical; to be made comical, it must be brought close.

Everything that makes us laugh is close at hand; therefore, all comical creativity works in a zone of maximal proximity. The idea is that the carnival brings the world close to us through its serious laughter:

> Laughter has the remarkable power of making an object come up close, of drawing it into a zone of crude contact where one can finger it familiarly on all sides, turn it upside down, inside out, peer at it from above and below, break open its external shell, look into its centre [!], doubt it, take it apart, dismember it, lay it bare and expose it, examine it freely and experiment with it. Laughter demolishes fear and piety before an object, before a world, making of it an object of familiar contact and thus clearing the ground for an absolutely free investigation of it. Laughter is a vital factor in laying down that prerequisite for fearlessness without which it would be impossible to approach the world realistically. As it draws an object to itself and makes it familiar, laughter delivers the object into the fearless hands of investigative experiment—both scientific and artistic—and into the hands of free experimental fantasy. (Bakhtin, 1981, p. 23)

As we can see, carnival involves a familiarization of the world through laughter. This is extremely important, says Bakhtin (1981, p. 23). In fact, "it is indispensable in making possible free, scientifically knowable, and artistically realistic creativity in European civilization" (Bakhtin, 1981).

This relates to the fact that during carnival, life is subject only to its own laws, the laws of its own freedom. A consequence is that carnival becomes a stage for insensible and irrational actions. Typical carnival characteristics are of the improvisational, experimental, explorative, aesthetic, and identifying sort. Also included in this are the freedom-based, the pretending, the transcendent, and the virtual, or the suspension of "reality."

Likewise, there is no footlight in carnival; in fact, footlights would destroy the carnival, just as the absence of footlights would destroy a theatrical performance (Bakhtin, 1984). Rather, the actors often get so engrossed in the event that while it lasts there is no other life outside it.

Because of their obvious sensuous character and their strong element of play, Bakhtin grants that carnival images closely resemble certain artistic forms, namely the spectacle. In turn, medieval spectacles often tended toward carnival folk culture, the culture of the marketplace, which to a certain extent became one of its components. However, ...

> the basic carnival nucleus of this culture is by no means a purely artistic form or spectacle and does not, generally speaking, belong to the sphere of art. Rather, it belongs to the borderline between art and life. In reality, it is life itself, but shaped to a certain pattern of play. (Bakhtin, 1984, p. 7)

Typical for the "between-space" (between art and life), which attracts people to participate, is the carnival's centrifugal force. Nothing compares to carnival when it comes to internal motivation and attraction.

A SHORT SUMMING UP OF BAKHTIN'S IDEAS

We see that Bakhtin's dialogue philosophy, in a fundamental way and not just as words, intersects with life itself; it does not exist without people and their actions and interactions, and never without a situated context. Bakhtin's use of voices is apparent here. A voice has meaning within a context and together with other voices. Thus, the voice of "I" can mean what "I" say, but only indirectly, since it is never solely responsible for its utterance and the meaning implied. Existence, too, becomes the event of co-being, which manifests itself in the form of a constant, ceaseless creation and exchange of meaning. Dialogue becomes a way for Bakhtin to define a human being's relation to another human being. In fact, dialogue is not just the basis for existence; it is also its goal and purpose. From this perspective, a human being uses language as a way not merely to express him-/herself, but also to communicate and to be in dialogue (Bakhtin, 1986b). Addressing the Other and/or the world through action requires being involved in a personal sense. Characteristically, answerability is the individual responsibility and obligation that leads to action by ourselves and also on behalf of others. Laughter is basic, not just to explore the world through masks and fantasy, but also as a way to bring reality close and vitalize our scientific and artistic actions. This process is an ongoing one, one that like Bakhtin's carnival creates threshold situations that characteristically involve joy and seriousness, ambivalence and paradoxes, harmony and dissonances, and so on.

Chapter 9

BAKHTIN'S IDEAS ON DIALOGUE TRANSPOSED TO RESPONSIVENESS IN MUSIC THERAPY IMPROVISATION

In this chapter, I start to merge my elaborations with Bakhtin's terminology through a reflective synthesis. This is the point in the book where my ideas increasingly take over from Bakhtin's.

My idea of responsiveness in music therapy improvisation associates with Bakhtin's dialogue as a combination of his real-life dialogue and a complexly organized cultural communication. A real-life dialogue is already associated in the log when Karla and Jakob face each other with their bodies and have a big djembe between them, on which both play and start taking turns. This is where the image of a café pops into Karla's head:

> *Karla finds herself standing outside the café looking through the window. On the inside, she sees two people drinking their lattes. They are turned toward each other—and focus their attention by asking: How are you …? How are we …? What shall we talk about? How shall we talk? They seem to have a lively conversation; their faces are expressive, alternately smiling and raising their eyebrows. They really make a lot of gestures, and one of them moves his arms a lot (Is he making some sort of a statement?). They are intensely present, but she wonders how well they really know each other. […] The coffee drinking seems to create a shape between them so that they know what to do with their hands. When one of them raises his/her cup, the other follows suit. The movements create a center between the two of them—. (see chapter 4)*

The image of the café shows how the music therapy situation could resemble a real-life dialogue. Both Jakob and Karla—without lattes but with a musical instrument (the djembe)—are in a position where both are ready to address the other, freely and openly, as in any lively conversation between two people.

The complexity connected to its culturally organized interaction relates to the improvisation's condensed and intensified way of shaping their interaction. The music therapy improvisation represents in this way something different from what most people think of as real-life dialogue. It is performed musically, not verbally, and is not as symmetrical as the image of the coffee drinkers in the café either. It involves a client, who needs help, and a music therapist, who is the "help expert." All together, these differences, along with several more, involve the typical music therapy way of cultivating and organizing the dialogical processes.

The narrative shows us that the responses in the music therapy improvisation between Jakob and Karla constitute a mix of musical and relational aspects. I will therefore refer to responses in music therapy improvisation as *musical-relational responses* in the following elaboration of Bakhtin's terms "dialogue" and "answerability."

I will return to some of the terms that I discussed in chapter 1, such as "action," "meaning," "improvisation," "ethics," and "aesthetics." My first issue is to discuss the book's most prominent term: "responsiveness."

RESPONSIVENESS IN MUSIC THERAPY IMPROVISATION

"Responsiveness" is a complex notion when we couple it with music therapy improvisation. It involves a multitude of aspects connected to actions and interactions in a social process where the players explore the various facets of music experience and the relationships formed through them (cf. Bruscia, 2014). Typically, client and therapist respond actively to each other's musical utterances in the here-and-now while at the same time searching for connections between them, but looking at such improvisation afterward shows how difficult it can be to find the "truth" inherent in it. It is thus perhaps time to renew our understanding of how we can embrace the intuitive and polyphonic aspects of music therapy improvisation so that we can modify and balance the creative process in an ethical and responsible sense (cf. Bruscia, 2014).

Two Levels of Responsiveness

Basically, I think that Bakhtin's ideas are transferable to responsiveness in music therapy improvisation on two levels. Lillis (2003), who speaks of dialogue, not responsiveness, inspires my outlining here.

Level 1 refers to meta-theoretical reflections, to responsiveness as given, and to the "nature" of improvisation in music therapy improvisation. This level reflects my intuitive feeling that improvisation in music therapy represents a unique and exciting—almost magnetic—way of exploring the creative being in the here-and-now. It reflects how the situated music therapy improvisation engages each player to act responsively to the other, to the situation, and to him-/herself.

Level 2 refers to responsiveness as a dialogical ideal, as something for which to struggle and work, against the forces of monologism. This level, I think, allows transference of Bakhtin's ideas to practical micro settings sometimes, such as the one between Jakob and Karla—but to many others as well. As an ideal, dialogue accepts that monologue happens and even is needed sometimes. It even questions whether there are situations when dialogism becomes too idealized.

Referring to both levels simultaneously in the following elaboration, I will present responsiveness as a mind-set, a dialogical mind-set, a consciously sought-after condition in the music therapist, something about which she can raise awareness and which, in turn, can inspire her personally and guide her in her improvisations. The mind-set requires that she resist the idea that she (always) knows what to expect from the client and that she is ready to be surprised by him. (I will return to my term "dialogical mind-set" in chapters 9, 11, and 15.)

Dialogical Responsiveness

Responsiveness, from the Bakhtinian perspective, is above all dialogical. Bakhtin, on a general level, would claim that dialogical responsiveness is essential to existence and to the human condition, because for him, life by its very nature is dialogical. Remember that Bakhtin (1984, p. 293) said: "To live means to participate in dialogue."

Responsiveness as Dialogue

My idea is that music therapy improvisation is a *living event* which is played out in which two (or more) "consciousnesses meet dialogically"

(Bakhtin, 1984, p. 72). *As* dialogue, responsiveness in music therapy improvisation is the process by which newer ways to respond, to mean, and to be can come into existence (cf. Lillis, 2003).

Therefore, and in the broadest understanding of "responsiveness"—if we accept music therapy improvisation to reflect a communicative human condition—every musical response in music therapy improvisation reflects life and being, in that it occasions new musical-relational responses in an unbroken chain of such responses. In this scenario, every musical-relational "utterance must be regarded as primarily a response to preceding utterances of the given sphere" (Bakhtin, 1986b, p. 1).

Responsiveness as a Multivoiced Activity

Responsiveness in the music therapy sphere becomes a multivoiced activity that is impressed with a plurality of consciousnesses. Who affects whom and what affects what at any moment is not easy to tell: It depends upon the individuals, their situation, and their actions. Their listening, too, is responsive—not just their playing. They prepare themselves to respond to what they are hearing, because none of them expects a passive understanding that duplicates only his or her own idea or music.

Responsiveness as Exploration

In a dialogical account of responsiveness, there are no preformed, orderly, and constant relations between the ideas and their music (Bakhtin, 1986b). There are only those responses that they develop or form as they attempt to express them musically and/or relationally to each other within the situation. For client and therapist, understanding the other's response means finding a "place" for it in the improvisation within the present context, while at the same time trying to capture what it does there and formulating a response to it.

Jakob and Karla Exploring Responsiveness

I find it meaningful here to draw parallels to the given sphere of the micro-level setting with Jakob and Karla. In the narrative, we learned that they had created a set of mutual response repertoires, such as vocalizing, strumming the guitar, hitting the djembe with a flat hand or scratching its skin with the fingers, or even an arm dancing in the air, and so forth. Jakob and Karla could refute, affirm, harmonize, supplement one another, and so on with this unique dialogical material.

If we use Bakhtin's ideas here, this suggests that they used their vocalizing, guitar strumming, and drum-playing to impose the "meaning" of their (musical) utterance on the other or to appropriate it by making it part of their own musical utterance with their dialogical material. Jakob and Karla even seemed to rely upon a (familiar) response from the other, as if they presupposed it to be "known." They somewhat took the other's response into account and expected another response that occasioned a further response in their improvisation.

The image of the expected ongoing chain of responses recalls a section of the logs written before The Guitar Excerpt starts, when Karla is hearing Jakob and his vocalizing as he is on his way to music therapy. During the improvisation, each of them listens to the other and plays with the other with an expectation of the other listening or playing while preparing a response, as an agreement, sympathy, objection, execution, and so forth (Stensæth, 2008).

The narrative shows how tendencies and feelings in the beginning were perhaps vague, chaotic, and diffusely distributed. Jakob's characteristic arm movements are examples of such. They could be understood as isolated utterances without interest and direction. As a sign, Jakob's arm movements receive meaning through the processes by which they are generated and used. When Karla understood Jakob's arm movements as if they were an initiation to a response coming from her, they became living carriers of meaning, as Bakhtin might have put it. There and then, Jakob and Karla opened themselves and permitted their communicative signs a degree of further specification.

In this way, they could negotiate with each other in ways that they found intelligible and legitimate. If they did not negotiate their musical-relational utterances in this way, there was no point in responding (cf. Shotter, 1992). Then the responsiveness in their music therapy improvisation would have collapsed.

Strangeness in the Responses—and Client and Therapist as Strangers

A response to be dialogical contains strangeness. For Bakhtin, there is no communication unless the Self lives through active understanding of the strange, also known as the Alter (Marková, 2003). Thus, there is no dialogical communication in the music therapy improvisation if

Jakob and Karla do not oppose one another through mutually experienced strangeness.

Every tone and every musical idea in their improvisation contains such strangeness. Typically, each of them tries to overpower the strangeness by imposing their meaning on the other and by making it part of their own playing and ideas.

Strangeness as Tension

The strangeness and the uncertainty creates tension. This tension does not "solve" the improvisation or end it, but instead creates direction and new interest in it. The tension is not bound to either of them, but actually exists between them, on a threshold between them and their musical actions. In this threshold, their actions and ideas vibrate, clash, judge, and evaluate one another.

This constant strife between the strangeness of their ideas makes their communication meaningful and essential to the human condition, which they are exploring together. The responsiveness would not be dialogical if the players were not opposed one to another through this mutually experienced strangeness.

The strangeness and the uncertainty of every music therapy situation creates tensions that uphold the participants' interest in each other and in their playing. This is essential for their interest in each other and the situation; their doings become "inter-essential" (as in a merging of the words "interest" and "essence").

Unfinalized Responses and Unfinalizable Individuals

Due to the strangeness involved in the responsiveness, we do not—and cannot—fully understand what is going on in the music therapy improvisation. We *try* to understand. We *try* to explain, through our theories and through our research, for example. However, and according to Bakhtin (1981), we cannot change the fact that responsiveness is unfinalizable because each one of us is unfinalized.

Jakob is always a riddle for Karla, and vice versa. They will always remain a riddle for each other. Matusov (2015) says that dialogue involves a constant expectation to be surprised by another person. It is "consciousness-as-it" rather than "consciousness as-you" (Matusov, 2015, p. 401; Matusov refers to Buber here). Therefore, Karla deals not just with the behavior of Jakob, but also with the mystery of him.

Matusov (2015) quotes a fellow Russian, Lobok, who argues that developmental psychology textbooks forget the most important thing about the child because they do not accept the child's uniqueness and her mystery. For Bakhtin, we cannot—and do not want to—live in the world where the other's consciousnesses is transparent and decoded to us. That would be the end of the world. The human being is always more than what we understand about him/her. This is always true, regardless of the age or the condition of the person.

Therefore, people are not mutually replaceable; they are unique. Each person therefore remains opaque, because each person is an unfinalized and ever-changing Universe (Matusov, 2015):

> People can be open to each other, while still remaining inexhaustible in their opaqueness. The more we engage with other people, the more we can learn and guess about their consciousness without ever fully "getting them" in width or depth. The more familiar they are, the richer people become to us in their puzzling opaqueness. (p. 400)

Jakob and Karla—just like every other human being, like you, the reader of this book, and me, the author—can therefore never completely understand each other either; we all become only partly satisfied with each other's responses. Dialogicality in responsiveness means accepting this (cf. Marková, 2003).

Comparisons with Other Philosophers

Mikhail Bakhtin versus Martin Buber and Emmanuel Levinas

We have heard that Bakhtin has much in common with other dialogue philosophers of his time. His resemblance to Martin Buber (1878–1965) and Emmanuel Levinas (1906–1995) is of special interest (Murray, 2009). The differences between them are perhaps not so large, but they are distinctive and deserve to be clarified in this context before I return to transferring Bakhtin's ideas to music therapy improvisation.

Bakhtin and Buber

Attunement to the attunement of the other is among the most important principles in dialogue philosophies. Dialogical mutuality for Buber is known in terms of I–Thou (Buber, 1992; Marková, 2003). This I–Thou relationship remains for Buber basically at the level of dialogue between human individuals, that is, at an interpersonal level.

For Bakhtin, however, there has to be something else in this world besides you and me (Marková, 2003). "Every individual lives 'in a world of others' words,'" Bakhtin said (1986b, p. 143). Bakhtin's view therefore ...

> redirects the focus on thinking and communication as a fusion of the minds or as something that always diminishes distances between people to dialogue as a communication in which the co-authors dispute, fight about ideas, and negotiate their antinomies in thinking. In dialogue, the participants confirm one another as co-authors of their ideas, and they also confirm their participation in social realities. (Marková, 2003, p. 256)

Bakhtin and Levinas

Levinas (1989, 1998) argues for the necessity of a primary sense, underlying all meaning, which provides the roots of an ethics beyond the differences of culture. He locates this sense in the original experience of the infinite Other, who, as the face of an abstract human being, calls the subject's very being into question.[13]

Levinas (1998) maintains that modern philosophy over-emphasizes the being as activity, as an engagement in the world rather than as an engagement with others. For him, engagement with the Other is moral, obligatory, and asymmetrical. Levinas emphasizes the separation between self and others and that human beings in their separation make moral demands. The self has no right to question what the other requires from him: His obligations to others are unlimited. This is fundamental and an a priori relation to the other, Levinas argues (1998); it is not ontology, but religion (e.g., Marková, 2003).

In Levinas's (1998) ethical approach, which has several similarities to Bakhtin's in that it emphasizes the I's responsibility toward Thou, communication seems to have the controlling power over the self: "The other calls upon me from a strange authority" (e.g., Marková, 2003). For Levinas, intersubjective communication can take place without words or gestures and just by facing the other. Levinas (1998) even doubts the notion of subjectivity. As he puts it, "The other takes precedence over me from the start; I am under allegiance to him" (p. 202). From this perspective, to be for the Other is almost to be without identity, Marková argues (2003), as if communication itself is a passivity of being.[14]

The Differences Between Bakhtin, Levinas, and Buber

From a Bakhtinian perspective, both Buber and Levinas become too antiindividualist in their dialogical approach (Marková, 2003). Marková (2003) finds that their approaches suggest a reduction of diverse positions of the self and other(s). For Bakhtin, intersubjectivity, understood as a fusion with the Other, is too narrow to account for the constitution of subjectivity. He says, "What would I have to gain if another were to fuse with me? [...] Let him rather remain outside me" (Bakhtin, 1986b, p. 78). Dialogical intersubjectivity is not about recognizing the other as the same, but "respecting the other as different and taking responsibility for this difference. [...] Dialogism means responding to alterity without negation or assimilation" (Peeren, in Kanellopoulos, 2011b, p. 124).

Bakhtin also makes a distinction between pure empathizing and active empathizing with the Other. Pure empathizing leads to the submerging of the self in the Other and viewing the world from the Other's perspective. Pure empathy erases the Other and leads to annihilation, to the loss of individuality, and to nonbeing, which is exactly what he does not want.

In contrast, active empathizing involves the struggle with Alter, with the strange. What arises from the struggle is something productive and new (Kanellopoulos, 2011b). This is Bakhtin's ideology. In fact, Bakhtin insists that a person has no internal sovereign territory and that he is wholly and always on the boundary with others. Communicating for him means to be "for another, through the other, for oneself" (Bakhtin, 1986b, p. 167). In other words, for Bakhtin, the limit of the Self is not I, but I in interrelationship with Other as separate personalities: "'I' *and* 'Thou'" (Marková, 2003, p. 256).

Moreover, living in a world with others is expressed by Bakhtin as co-authorship rather than intersubjectivity: Co-authorship demands evaluation of the Other, struggle with the Other, and judgment of the message of the Other, and this creates natural tension. Through the tension, the Self is not attempting to fuse with the Other but, instead, to set his own position and to assimilate strangeness.

Marková (2003) suggests that the capacity of the human mind to conceive, create, and communicate about social realities in terms of the Alter must complement intersubjectivity in conceptualizations of subjectivity in a Bakhtinian perspective. Therefore, for Bakhtin, all symbolic activity of humans is founded on (active) dialogue between different minds expressing multitudes of multivoiced meanings (Marková, 2003).

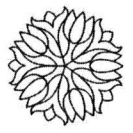

Chapter 10

BAKHTIN'S IDEAS ON ANSWERABILITY, TRANSPOSED TO RESPONSIVENESS IN MUSIC THERAPY IMPROVISATION

Bakhtin's ideas on dialogue, transposed to responsiveness in music therapy improvisation, create a close link to this chapter, which involves my transposing of his term "answerability." I will start with an abstract that will take us from dialogue to answerability.

In a Bakhtinian perspective, responsiveness in music therapy improvisation requires active, face-to-face, musical-relational responding from both client and therapist, not in the sense of a fusion of their minds, but as engaging in the co-authorship of the musical improvisation. In their playing, Jakob and Karla are both "dialogically laden" with the musical "traces" of each other (Bakhtin, 1984, p. 287), but as individuals, they will always remain outside each other. They might feel that they share the music and the improvisation, but they do not necessarily experience the same thing. In a sense, their inner lives are moved out and into the improvisational threshold between them. For their actions to become dialogical, they must actively approach the threshold together. The improvisation is a common task: One of them is not enough. Responsiveness takes the two of them; in fact, it depends upon both of them to create a collective musical-relational sculpting that they can constantly negotiate. This is an important point in Bakhtin's philosophy: Each of them is there for the other and, through the other (and through their musical improvisation), for themselves. This is a commitment that is part of their responsibility, in their being in the world. We are talking about answerability.

Responsiveness and Answerability

For Bakhtin, dialogicality implies contract: responsiveness *and* responsibility. Acts performed by client and therapist in music therapy are therefore intentional, but for them to be effective, they require personal commitment and responsibility (Marková, 2003). There can be no music, no improvisation, no tone, no utterance, and no rhythm without a player. There can be no music without a history, either, and there can be no music without the Self. On the contrary, the loss of commitment to the music and to the playing could result in the player's loss of Self-identity and authenticity.

Thus, responsiveness in music therapy improvisation requires that both client and therapist feel personally obligated to act. Only in this way can they be mutually answerable toward each other. I argue that the music (especially performed as improvisation) engages Jakob and Karla so that they feel obligated to act. The music therapist's willingness to "musicalize" (my word) Jakob's actions (e.g., his arm movements) is vital for Jakob's obligation. I also argue that the relation to Other and his/her actions engage each of them so that they feel obligated to act.

Panagiotis Kanellopoulos on the "Oughtness" to Act

My idea of a sense of an "oughtness" to act stems from Panagiotis A. Kanellopoulos (2011a), who refers to Bakhtin's answerability in improvisation in music education. He wants to get away from the (traditional) apprehension of musical improvisation as simple speeded-up composing or as script-*less* performing, and the "domination of psychological theorizing of improvisation as a form of skill-based expertise" (Kanellopoulos, 2011b, p. 131):

> Instead, we need to reshape our understanding of the social nature of the improvisation experience: by emphasizing unfinalizability (of both music and selves) and the impossibility for a single consciousness to gain privileged access to truth, it leads to the search for "a dialogic sense of truth [which] manifests unfinalizability by existing in the 'threshold' of several interacting consciousnesses, a 'plurality' of 'unmerged voices.'" [Kanellopoulos, 2011a; Kanellopoulos refers here to quotes in Shotter's (1992) comparisons of Bakhtin and Billig]

Kanellopoulos sees improvisation as a mode of musical practice that requires the development of a particular attitude of consciousness, as a way of delving into music-making which transforms the traditional understanding in the way that it redefines musical aesthetics and its relation to agency, expression, and the sociality of music. In his picture, musical improvisation is a public musical space that is marked by the absence of fear, where exploration of musical freedom is pursued, and where everything might happen but not anything goes (Kanellopoulos, 2011a).

Further on, Kanellopoulos says that one could draw an analogy between the experience of reading a novel and creating and/or attending a musical improvisation since both share a "specific 'impulse to continue' (what will happen next?) and the 'impulse to end' (how will it end?)" (cf. Bakhtin, 1981, p. 32).

Kanellopoulos uses the term "dialogic improvisation" to emphasize that the improvisation involves the essential unfinalizability of musical selves and musical interactions. Dialogic improvisation constitutes …

> a context which both enables and obliges the participants to develop a sense of responsibility with respect to the pursuit of free musical thinking, guarding the moment of improvisation as a precious, distinct moment of invention (Kanellopoulos, 2011a, p. 99).

In this distinct moment of invention, the players will feel an obligation to play. This in turn creates an improvisational attitude that implies "obligation," or "oughtness," to let go in the playing (Kanellopoulos, 2011a):

> The attitude developed by the improviser is marked by a sense of "obligation" to *surrender* to the music created, both accepting the direction taken each time and *deciding* upon the course of this direction (Kanellopoulos, 2011a, p. 95, author's italics).

This view suggests that the distinctiveness of improvisation lies in its potential to create and cultivate a particular quality of attention to the unfolding present of musical moments, in its particular understanding of "the ought" (Kanellopoulos, 2011a).

Kanellopoulos's perspective is relevant for music therapy, too. In the case of Karla and Jakob, for example, it suggests that they sense this type of "ought" when they are experiencing how to pursue the unknown in their improvisation. The "ought" is not enforced by something beyond the immediate act of their improvisation. Instead, within the moment of improvisation, and while they both are co-authoring it together, Jakob and Karla decide the direction of their musical improvisation. Then they invent ideas, which are repeated, developed, abandoned, deconstructed. All this leads them to new knowledge of the inherent openness and indeterminacy of their improvisation (cf. Kanellopoulos, 2011a).

The "Ought" in Music Therapy Improvisation

In music therapy improvisation, and as a variation of the Kanellopoulos perspective, the music therapy improvisation creates a type of obligation that is caused not only by the music, but also by their relation and its musicalized actions together, as one.

The Musical-Relational "Ought" Exemplified with Jakob and Karla

As we have seen in the narrative, Karla actively approaches Jakob face-to-face. She actively "reads" him: his actions, gestures, and desires. Jakob, too, faces Karla, although not as directly all the time (he moves his face away every now and then). When Jakob starts to move his body (his arms, in particular), he is vitalized and raises his arms into the air. In this way, he shows that he feels "the ought" to continue.

Karla immediately reads his arm movements as music, as musicalized actions to her playing and as responses from him to her. She then responds to him by giving a musical shape to whatever utterances he makes. When he raises his arms into the air, as in a dance, she makes flamenco-like rallentandos on the guitar to accompany his arm-dancing. By so doing, she adds her semantic and expressive intention to his arm movements to her music.

Jakob, for his part, responds to her music-making by moving his arms in an even more dancelike way. Through this, he shows that he has a sense that she understands his arm movements as musical utterances and that he can use his arms to respond musically to Karla and collaborate actively in their collective music-making. In this way, he, too, actively adds his semantic and expressive intention to whatever she does.

They create a type of improvisation that engages them both in the moment; they surrender to it and accept the direction that it takes each time. I therefore advocate for a type of "musical-relational obligation." This is also an "ought" that creates an impulse to continue (e.g., what will happen next?) and an impulse to end (e.g., how will it end?). It is an "ought" where the Other's strangeness (the Alter) and the musical freedom create a magnetic and irresistible driving force in them to want the improvisation to continue. They both feel responsible to act upon the other in their creative musical-relational way.

Music as the Spark of a Musical-Relational Answerability

Behind the idea that the musical improvisation creates the feeling of "obligation" to surrender is the point that the music also offers a suitable agent that provides client and therapist with a form with which they can shape their dramaturgy (cf. Kruse, 2016; see chapter 1).

With the help of music, Karla can musicalize Jakob's arm movements and include them in their interaction. The music also helps Jakob, because it arouses him to act and move his arms, which, in turn, provides a dialogical repertoire for his participation. For him, as someone who cannot improvise musically in the same way as other musicians, this is crucial: The musical-relational improvisation creates a way for him to participate creatively, collectively, and answerably with himself, the Other, and "the world."

Their unique way of creating the musical-relational improvisation becomes the way that Jakob and Karla communicate. It represents their dialect; it is their "music-relation-ness" (my word, i.e., heteroglossia as different speech-ness; see chapter 8). The narrative therefore not only describes how they "speak" with each other in a specific type of discourse, but also shows how their obligation to act emerges from within the situation:

> The obligation to act freely is created out of the conception of improvisation that emerges out of a practice and cultivates a particular attitude toward the making of music. The musician's acts are answerable to nothing and to no one but to the density of immersion to the moment of invention, to the decision to search for musical freedom. This immersion to the moment is the outcome of the performative

irrevocability of improvisation. Within the act of improvisation, this experience of the irrevocability of a musical *future* that keeps becoming musical past should be seen as closely related to the emergence of the musician's responsibility to cultivate musical freedom. (Kanellopoulos, 2011a, p. 95, author's italics)

Jakob and Karla might experience their improvisation as a mode of musical practice that demands them to value the immediacy of each moment, as a moment they want to expand and continue, so that it creates newer ways for them to mean and to be. Their inventions are not given. They are not merely expressing Jakob's ideas or feelings or Karla's ideas or feelings. Instead, they lie on the threshold before "the fundamental plurality of unmerged consciousnesses" (Bakhtin, 1984, p. 9). This, to me, is the nature of responsiveness in music therapy improvisation. The task is simply that of understanding, which means finding connections in their doings.

It is only their immersion in the moment that each one of them (the Self) is answerable *for*. Both of them are answerable *to* the responsiveness. We cannot change this, and therefore we are all ethically obliged to respond:

We are responsible in the sense that we are *compelled* to respond, we cannot choose but to give the world an answer, each one of us occupies a place in existence that is uniquely ours; but far from being a privilege, far from having what Bakhtin calls an alibi in existence, the uniqueness of the place I occupy in existence is, in its deepest sense of the word, an answerability: in that place only I am addressed by the world, since only I am in it. Moreover, we must keep on forming responses as long as we live. (Holquist, 1990, pp. 29–30)

Being answerable *to* responsiveness, Karla of course has another responsibility, too—one that is of a professional kind.

THE MUSIC THERAPIST'S RESPONSIBILITY

Karla's responsibility, in a Bakhtinian perspective, is complex. As Emerson (2000) describes it, responsibility involves so much:

Bakhtin's responsibility must presume a series of miraculous balances. There must be outsideness but not aloneness; a vulnerable openness to participation but at the same time autonomy and indifference to critical assault or personal rejection; a full reserve of "aesthetic love" but combined with a willingness to be more lover than beloved. I can never demand from another person the specific content I think I need. (p. 284)

The therapist's professional responsibility is different from her responsibility as a person. However, she is always personally answerable to herself and her place in the world, even in professional settings. Therefore, she can try—ideally—to enter the music therapy improvisation with a genuine personal interest. She might, both personally and professionally, "other" herself to the response and to the unknown within the situation. By pursuing the unknown and sustaining the search for it, in the music, in the client, in herself, in aesthetic love, she sustains an awareness of the unfinalizability of responsiveness.

Answerability in a Professional Sense

Bakhtin's dialogical idea that people must "keep on forming responses as long as we live" (see the previous citation by Holquist) is interesting for the music therapist, on both a personal level as well as a professional level. On a professional level, it gives her a reason for being a music therapist: It suggests that doing music therapy is an ethically answerable act.

Answerability in a Personal Sense

However, the therapist can never escape from her personal answerability. Approaching the client actively and face-to-face, with the intention of immersing in the moment with him and in his musical-relational utterances, is something through which she responds to the world and *her* place in it. It is a personal answerable act. In this way, she can respond to the situation both personally and professionally by confirming Jakob's existence and allowing him to confirm her existence.

For Jakob to come forth, Karla's obligation is crucial: Karla, both professionally and personally, supports Jakob in searching for his own personal voice, his individual voice, his being in the world, which belongs to the larger dialogical context of which we are all part (cf. Matusov, 2009).

Obviously, Jakob's actions and utterances are different from the ordinary everyday communication that most of us know. He manifests himself by vocalizing and moving his body—in particular, his arms. He needs Karla to "read him" and approach his arm movements as something that goes beyond the ability to move a limb. This is not possible if she does not immerse herself in the musical-relational improvisation with authenticity and a sense of oughtness through which she sees him—like herself—as an unfinalized Alter.

Stepping Outside and Reflect-in-Action

Preferably, Karla should fuse her personal responsibility with her professional responsibility. The professional responsibility requires that she reflects-in-action (cf. Schön, 1983), which she can do by stepping outside the immersion of the moment. Obviously, this is taking a step out of dialogue, too. Stepping aside and away from the situation like this involves monologue, or what Kanellopoulos (2011a) calls "outsideness" (p. 100). In using the concept of outsideness in the context of the improvisation process, Kanellopoulos (2011b) emphasizes two aspects:

> The first relates to the requirement that the player(s)' actions and attention allow for reflection which might be seen as an instance of "exercising a surplus of vision with respect to the event" and the second to the "participatory (oriented toward another consciousness, response-worthy)" nature of improvisation.[15] (p. 124)

"Outsideness," in my context, refers to Karla's ability to "see" her own actions from a certain distance. The oughtness is still the guiding force, but "stepping out" is a movement of the mind, an act of looking at what she is doing from a certain distance (Kanellopoulos, 2011b). Stepping out functions as a means of "creating temporary finalizations" (Kanellopoulos, 2011a, p. 99).

Without the creation of temporary finalizations like this, the continuity of the improvisation experience would not even be possible (Kanellopoulos, 2011a). Therefore, stepping out requires openness from her, an openness that demands that decisions are taken and that their consequences become part of the musical-relational playing in which they both assume authorship of their actions, "acting as if they were the only ones that could have been made" (Kanellopoulos, 2011a, p. 99).

Being immersed in the musical improvisation therefore does not entirely exclude Karla from active evaluation of the process. Through a concurrent struggle to step outside what she is doing, trying to see it from afar, she can still take part in the here-and-now, as long as her mind-set maintains being dialogical. Stepping out does not change anything. Her comprehension of the situation is still not final; rather, it is transformed but never fully created from scratch (cf. Matusov, 2015).

Stepping out allows her to reflect-in-action. Such reflection-in-action is "action present." Schön (1983) describes this as reflecting on the incident while it can still benefit that situation rather than reflecting in the future on how you would have done or would do things differently. This is a useful tool to use in disciplines where the professional has to react to an event at the time it occurs, not having the luxury of being able to think about what happened and making changes at a later time. This process is described by Schön (1983) in this way:

> When someone reflects-in-action, he becomes a researcher in the practice context. He is not dependent on the categories or established theory and technique, but constructs a new theory of the unique case.[16] (p. 68)

Searching for (Dialogical) Meaning

Bakhtin defined dialogical meaning-making as a dialogical relationship between the genuine, personal, authentic question of one person seeking information and the serious reply by another person in a never-ending dialogue. Matusov paraphrases a famous quote about culture from Bakhtin when suggesting that "meaning does not have internal territory" (Matusov, 2009, p. 120).

This suggests that Karla's search for meaning is rooted in the dialogical responsiveness in which both she and Jakob participate. The meaning is fleeting (cf. Aksnes & Ruud, 2008; see chapter 1). It is something that they both continuously explore, something they try to find a place for as they immerse in their playing. Because they can (never) completely understand each other, Jakob and Karla become only partly satisfied with each other's responses.

Meaning is placed on the threshold, somewhere between them and their minds. Just as the meaning cannot be placed in Karla's consciousness alone (unified and closed in itself), it gives rise to new meanings. Thus, if Karla's perception of the music therapy improvisation falls completely out of dialogue, it enters systemic cognition, which is essentially impersonal (Matusov, 2009). This is not what Bakhtin wants; it is not what I want either. Therefore, meaning is possible to find, but only when the players are being open-minded, subjective and biased (Matusov, 2015, p. 409), and personally engaged.

Helping the Client Becoming Response-able

Responsiveness, then, requires shared responsibility for the music-making. Karla's responsibility within the improvisation is cultivated by the immediacy of her decision-making (cf. Kanellopoulos, 2011a). By stepping outside (in her mind) without stepping out of the process, she looks for ways in which she might transfer them into responsive material so that they fit into something they can share and develop further together. To put it simply, the therapist—and to play with words again—is respons*ible* for making the client becoming response-*able*.

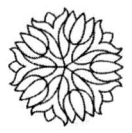

Chapter 11

"WE:" A COMMUNITY OF MUSIC THERAPY IMPROVISATION

This chapter discusses how responsiveness in music therapy improvisation could create the feeling of a community, a "We." This perspective is inspired by Eugene Matusov (2009, 2011), and merges my transposing of insights from Bakhtin's dialogue and answerability in chapters 9 and 10. I will again materialze my ideas by referring to the narrative between Jakob and Karla.

A COMMUNITY OF MUSIC THERAPY IMPROVISATION

Matusov (2009, 2010, 2011), in his dialogical pedagogy, says that learning is an issue that involves all of the people in the learning process, both the teacher and the pupil. Together, they create a *community of learning* (Matusov, 2009, 2011). Through the community, the learning becomes an ongoing, unfinalizable, and polyphonic project mediated not just by consensus and agreement but also by dissonances and disagreement by those who participate, Matusov claims.

I suggest a similar label for the music therapy improvisation: *a community of music therapy improvisation*. My label suggests that optimizing the client's health (e.g., Bruscia, 2014) is not the therapist's project alone. It is certainly not the client's project either. Instead, it is a joint project that requires that they both make efforts to establish responsiveness.[17] What does this imply for the case of Jakob and Karla?

A Community of Improvisation for Jakob and Karla

First, as a community of music therapy improvisation, Karla, the music therapist, cannot help Jakob to accomplish a goal that he could not otherwise accomplish on his own. Karla must first of all see herself and Jakob as a *We*, as in Schütz's We (see chapter 1), as a mutually tuning-in relationship that originates in the possibility of living together simultaneously not only within a specific musical-relational tune, but also as a community of improvisers who both can learn, develop, and change. This is basic.

Second, a community of music therapy improvisation would mean that Karla could not play for herself or simply together with Jakob. He, the client, would not need Karla solely to accompany him musically or play along with him. Because his playing cannot be heard and understood as an isolated unit, Jakob in fact needs Karla to influence him and his music in an inescapably intertwined way.

Third, as a community of music therapy improvisation, they both need the other to become themselves. Each utterance, each single tone that they play does not exist inside them. Rather, this exists on the threshold between them. Karla's drum-playing becomes Jakob's, which it does when it is populated with *their* musical accent and adapted to *their* musical semantic and expressive intention. Similarly, Jakob's arm movement becomes Karla's when both of them experience it as *their* musical-relational theme. Its identity belongs to both of them: It is "dialogized." This is a foundation for a community of music therapy improvisation.

Defining a Dialogical Agency in Each Other

This all must not be understood as if Karla can play only for Jakob and not for herself. Empathizing totally with Jakob and his music so much that she silences her own voice would be a misunderstanding. The point is that they both need each other to define a *dialogical agency* in each other (e.g., Matusov, 2009). Their drum-playing or arm movement, to become a sound of *their* music-making, is always a medium for negotiation; it is always half–someone else's, to borrow Bakhtin's words again. "Someone else's" is that of either the other (sitting) opposite or of other consciousnesses we possibly could sense as being present (such as those of theorists, composers, or musicians who influence our music or relatives or friends who inspire us personally). As persons, Jakob and

Karla can never be fully revealed (or fully known in the world, as Bakhtin says) without the voice of the Other.

Monological Aspects

Is a dialogical mind-set and the idea of a community of music therapy improvisation always required in practical situations as described in the narrative with Jakob and Karla? Probably it is not possible for Karla to maintain an optimal engagement with Jakob at all times (cf. Matusov, 2001, 2009). Therefore, not all therapy requires dialogue mediation. The dialogical mind-set is an ideal, and sometimes a more monological mediation is even appropriate. By themselves, dialogical and monological mediations are neither good nor bad. In fact, it can be difficult to discern between monologue and dialogue. They both constitute aspects of any discourse.

In the discourses, however, one dominates over the other. To learn how to play a scale on an instrument, to learn a skill, for example, or to understand the playing as a final response and not a stream of many possible utterances, creates monologue. When the therapist's response does not reflect the other's expressions—or the qualities in her expressions—the mediation is monological.

Orchestration of dialogue, says Matusov (1996), involves mediation of issues of exclusion involving the players' access to and comfort in the dialogue and its fragmentation. When the purpose is to promote, support, and deepen the dialogue, the mediation even becomes polyphonic (Matusov, 1996).

Dialogue and Monologue as Complementary Aspects

Matusov (2009) suggests dialogue and monologue as complementary and co-existent, as two inherent aspects of human consciousness that complement each other: "Monologicity is impossible without a strong sense of recognition and acceptance by others and thus is shaped by dialogicity" (p. 132). The problem with monologism is not that it is closed, but that it presents itself as a bearer of a truth that has not been the result of co-authorship.

Creating a dialogical context for the musical improvisation between Jakob and Karla urges them both to create links between each concrete response (e.g., Jakob's arm movements), the historical depths from which it emerges, and the sociality of its future responses.

Probing (exploring) and questioning their sources becomes a context for therapy. The dialogical ideal is thus that responsiveness in music therapy improvisation creates a We-community in which both Jakob and Karla can act answerably. Together they create something unique; they build a type of musical togetherness that creates bonding and belonging between them but also is one in which each of them feels that they can be who they are (cf. Stensæth & Næss, 2013).[18]

Vulnerable Relations and Face-to-Face Positioning

Practicing a philosophy of a community of music therapy improvisation requires that the music therapist has a deep personal care about and commitment to her client. This commitment is based on sympathy, attachment, and compassion. This is even more important in vulnerable relations (Tønsberg, 2010), such as in music therapy settings with a client like Jakob, who has severe physical and mental handicaps, and a therapist like Karla, who possesses (much) power. Their relationship is vulnerable because it creates greater risks for misunderstanding and therefore also dialogical collapse.

Vulnerable relations could therefore create a poor basis for dialogue, and one might ask if Bakhtin's ideas on dialogue are transferable to them at all. Several researchers within the field of music therapy advocate for the use of dialogue philosophy, especially in therapy settings that include vulnerable relations (Garred, 2004; Horgen, 2010; Stensæth, 2008, 2010; Trondalen, 2016; Tønsberg, 2010). They suggest that a dialogical ideal (which is embedded in my term "dialogical mind-set") is even urgent in these relations (Garred, 2004; Horgen, 2010; Stensæth, 2008, 2010; Trondalen, 2016; Tønsberg, 2010) due to the risk of the misuse of power.

Along with Tønsberg (2010), I believe that dialogue is important to struggle for in the music therapy improvisation. Bakhtin's (and Levinas's) dialogical face-to-face positioning is both desirable and necessary, although it is risky and challenging. It requires above all that the therapist, who is the one with the most power in the relationship, possess an ethical and aesthetical awareness about her role.

Ethical Aspects in Vulnerable Relationships

To activate a dialogical agency in each other, Karla and Jakob must experience whatever is happening between them as mutually shared.

Only in this way can she see his resources and potentials and not his limitations and abnormal expressions. Ethically, a face-to-face positioning would first require that each of them listen openly to the voice of the other.

Obviously, Karla's role is different from Jakob's in this respect. She must first (a) recognize Jakob's (active and passive) participation in Being, and then (b) see his uniqueness as given but simultaneously as one that exists only to the degree to which she can actualize it (cf. Bakhtin, 1986b). Therefore, it is when Karla actually sees herself as the potential Other for Jakob that she proves how dialogue first of all requires two minds, not the same experiences (Stensæth, 2010).

Responsiveness as a Human Capacity

Dialogue in this perspective is seen as the (inherent) "capacity of the human mind to conceive, create, and communicate about social reality in terms of the Alter" (Marková, in Tønsberg, 2010, p. 46). Such an understanding unifies with Bakhtin's in that it views dialogue only in relation to other human beings and in the notion that we are all born with a dialogical mind, which is reflected by other people's minds. Most of all, this kind of posture calls for compassion and care, in just the way a mother or a father intuitively would relate to her/his infant (cf. communicative musicality).

Being a "Close Other"

For Karla to position herself face-to-face with Jakob may seem obvious and simple, but in fact it can be extremely complex and challenging in a vulnerable relationship like theirs. Horgen (2010) says that practicing ethics in vulnerable relationships demands that someone take the role of the "close other" and that the Other actually experience her as close. A close other is one who relates seriously and with sympathy, attachment, and compassion to all possible communicative signals from the Other.[19]

Transferring this perspective to the narrative, this suggests that Karla, as the therapist, should constrain herself to leave space for Jakob, the client. This is possible only if she lets go and puts herself into play for him.

To Doubt One's Own Voice

To do so, she must doubt (not forget) her own voice and let his voice influence her. Doubting her own voice would imply that she doubts what she knows, such as knowledge and theories, imaginations, prejudices, wishes, goals, experiences, and so forth. This doubting is necessary to welcome Jakob and his actions and to focus on whatever he has on his mind.

We have already seen in the narrative how Karla relates to his utterances (a spastic movement, a tension, or an involuntary or accidental body movement) that were perhaps not intended as dialogue. As the therapist, and to create material for dialogue, she might, however, listen to them as if they were *dialogically intended*.

Ulla Holck on Expectation

This recalls music therapist Holck (2004), who created the term "interaction themes" to cover what is going on in the musical improvisation in therapy situations with children with severe handicaps. Holck finds that the function of the interaction themes is to promote *expectations* regarding the interaction, which this author thinks is the very spark of any dialogical agency.

For the interaction to create expectation in a Bakhtinian picture involves something more than the repetition of an intention or the establishment of a ritual. It requires socially spontaneous (prereflective) interactions that unfold in time within the situation where their intention is (still) indefinite (cf. Østerberg, 1993; see chapter 2). This type of expectation contains both the known and the unknown, uncertainty and openness, which are needed for the players to create further interest in each other and their development of new interaction themes. Expectation is a label that one interaction theme is never final; it belongs to a chain of interaction themes.

An Ethical and Loving Responsiveness

In a community of music therapy improvisation, offering a loving, engaging, and emotionally co-living sense of being there for the client is not enough for the therapist. She needs him, the client, for her life to become valuable, "not in the category of the I, but in the category of the Other, as the life of another person, another I" (Bakhtin, 1986b, pp.

79–82). She in fact needs him to avoid losing herself (to subjectivity).

Ethically, this (dialogical ideal) means that, next to committing herself to the situation and immersing herself in the music-making (cf. Kanellopoulos, 2011a, 2011b) with the client (and his strangeness, e.g., the Other as Alter), responsiveness must become essential for her own sake, for the sake of her identity, and from her position as an "I." Matusov (2015) explains this as follows:

> People essentially need each other, not because they can become more powerful in fulfilling their own desires and can do together more than they can do alone. People essentially need each other not because they need to consume the consciousnesses of the others as much as possible. No. Rather, I argue, people need each other because they are lonely otherwise and need the others as their interlocutors whom they never fully understand and whose consciousness is unique and will always remain unique, opaque, and incomprehensible. (p. 400)

In my understanding, Bakhtin approaches a view here where he sees the intersubjective relationship as aesthetic and loving. This must not be understood as a simple matter of everyday encounters between two people. Instead, it is an extraordinary encounter, one that Hirschkop (1990, p. 60, referring to Bakhtin) describes as a "free and unmotivated (that is, disinterested) affirmation of the value of another." Out of this perspective emerges an aspect that we could understand as Bakhtin's ethics of aesthetics.

An Aesthetical Awareness in the I–You Relation

Børtnes (2001) writes about the aesthetical aspects of Bakhtin's "dialogue." He says that to relate to the Other in a dialogical sense calls for an aesthetical awareness in the I–You relation. In this relation, the You and the I face each other as subjects. Børtnes thinks that in the dialogue between this I and You, the I appears not just as a random individual who is put there for the occasion, but as a loving and doubting personality (Børtnes, 2001, p. 103; see also Horgen, 2010). This view contradicts a cognitive awareness through which the Other becomes (solely) an object for learning, therapy, or research.

Horgen (2010) picks up on Børtnes's writing and suggests that in therapy with vulnerable relationships, a goal for the therapist's aesthetical awareness is to become a true You, who hears, sees, and loves the Other while doubting the I. For a therapist, this perspective involves developing a loving, engaging, and "emotionally co-living" sense of being there for the Other (Horgen, 2010, p. 13).

Taking the Position of a Participant, not a Spectator

To explain the significance of such aesthetical awareness in music therapy improvisation, music therapy researcher Gro E. H. Tønsberg compares the positions taken by a participant with the position of a spectator of art: When Da Vinci's famous painting of Mona Lisa arouses our curiosity and fantasy, we start imagining what her mystic smile could possibly mean. At the moment when we get engaged in creating the scenario behind the smile, we take the position of a participant and step away from being in the position of a spectator (Tønsberg, 2010, who here refers to Nafstad, the psychologist).

In the same way, says Tønsberg, we need to take the position of a participant in the life of the Other, not that of a spectator. Tønsberg (2010) suggests that a participant position relative to the Mona Lisa painting shows how aesthetic forms of expression are dialogical in nature. Perhaps this image is a simple but good illustration of another dialogical premise in musical improvisation in vulnerable relations?

Music as an Aesthetical Agent

Aesthetics in Bakhtin's picture brings us back to the creative process of music therapy improvisation (and its relationship to art, life, and ethics). As a music therapist, this author has often felt that the aesthetics of music becomes an agent that takes part in the improvisation on its own terms, in the sense that the experience of the music unifies with the experience of the client. Aigen (1991), the music therapist, describes something similar:

> What is occurring is that I am becoming aware of the music as a unique manifestation of the client. The duality of person and act disintegrates, and I experience the music as the person, not as the symbol or representation. I am living in the music in the same way as I am perceiving the client within his or her music, and while words can be used to later

> describe what occurred, the entire process takes place on a nonverbal, musical level. (p. 236)

Garred (2004, 2006), by transferring Buber's philosophy on I and You to music therapy, is perhaps more precise in his explanation when he points out that a musical improvisation involves a human relationship *caused by the music*. He suggests that this relationship behaves differently from other relations. The musical relationship in general seems to be more vital and emotional and includes evidentially more bodily expressions than many other types of relations (without music). I add up all of the aspects into one aspect and suggest that it is musical-relational (Stensæth, 2008). To add the musical-relational aesthetics to Bakhtin's meta-perspective, it must be understood as sociocultural and situated.

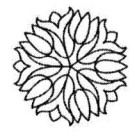

Chapter 12

BAKHTIN'S IDEAS ON CARNIVAL, TRANSPOSED TO RESPONSIVENESS IN MUSIC THERAPY IMPROVISATION

Bakhtin's term "carnival" belongs to a sphere different from that of his dialogue. It is of another character than dialogue and its existential ideals, especially because it recognizes the value and importance of bodily involvement and collectivity, of laughter and play. Carnival will be referred to in this chapter as a metaphor for people's need to get in contact with these aspects of life. I will also creatively return to the narrative as real-life events and include aspects of Steinsholt's play philosophy to describe my points. This part of the book is where my ideas are furthest removed from Bakhtin's meta-perspective.

CARNIVAL AND IMPROVISATION

The Need for Carnival for Jakob and Karla

When life is difficult, for example, when we have adverse health conditions—or, perhaps, *particularly* in such times—we need to feel that we are vitally present in own life, with our bodies and with both joy and ridicule. Many people, like Jakob, do not have easy access to the types of experiences that the carnival represents.

I argue that music therapy and the improvisational approach is important because it might engage people in carnival-like experiences. Jakob and Karla's improvisation affords—as carnival—a way for them to participate in life with serious laughter, meaningful chaos, and so forth. In this light, Jakob and Karla's narrative tells a story about a practice that provides another type of act, representing "a plane equal to contemporary life" (cf. Bakhtin, 1981, p. 21).

Carnival as Democracy

Jakob and Karla's improvisation can be seen as a critique of the monologization of the human experience that we might perceive through dominant scientific and political theories. I argue that music therapy improvisation, like carnival, represents a radical and anti-authoritative communication event. In this sense, it is a criticism of society's high and low categories of people, art, communication. Democracy, in fact, needs the depth offered by activities like music therapy improvisation. In this picture, improvisation in music therapy represents a way of creating and cultivating local democratic micro-cultures.

In this way, carnival shows how the music therapy improvisation might become an emancipating activity wherein client and therapist can experiment with meaning and invest their fantasies. The improvisation becomes a way for them, to borrow the words of Bruscia (2014, p. 130), to "develop creativity, expressive freedom, playfulness, with various degrees of structure" in which they can try out new ways of being. Bakhtin's perspective on carnival is helpful to modify and balance the creative process in music therapy improvisation in an ethical and a responsible sense. This is a basis for music therapists in their work to optimize people's health.

Carnival Characteristics

Several characteristics of Bakhtin's carnival have been helpful in my exploration of music therapy improvisation as a type of democratization process:
- The first characteristic is that carnival creates a "place" for familiar and free interaction between people, one that brings people together and encourages unlikely collaboration.
- Another characteristic is that carnival welcomes unacceptable behavior and that its formats allow "everything," because carnival contains strange and odd actions and exploration of creative and theatrical expressions. (I like, for example, to think of music as masks through which client and therapist can explore each other in creative ways.)
- Yet a third characteristic, and perhaps one of its most essential,

is carnival's unique attraction. This attraction, which Bakhtin refers to as carnival's centrifugal forces, explains why people want to take part and, from this, how they unfold freely, uninhibited and with joy and desire. The narrative is an illustration of this.

These characteristics will turn up in different forms throughout the chapter.

KJETIL STEINSHOLT'S CARNIVAL: CARNIVAL AS PLAY

Steinsholt has inspired my adoption of carnival to music therapy improvisation, and he uses Bakhtin's carnival as a metaphor for his thoughts on play. He suggests that play, rather than being an activity connected to areas such as education and development, involves a "carnival lifestyle." Play is where the children enter the spectacle and come together "to live the carnival life" (Steinsholt, 1998):

> They [the children] can move to and fro, in and out of the spectacle; they can tease, imitate, and be ridiculous; they can get into verbal fights and exaggerate their own body movements and make fun of the grown-ups' stories about the world. (p. 34, my translation)

Play, just like Bakhtin's carnival, implies no footlight or any distinction between actors and spectators. Steinsholt thinks that carnival reveals that play is essentially freedom-based (Steinsholt, 1998). It is a place where the children freely and willingly come and go. Most important, according to Steinsholt: Bakhtin's carnival, like play, represents a chance for the children's voices to be heard.

A World Upside Down

Also typical is that life is turned upside down for a while in (intense) play; the insensible is allowed, and fragments, repetitions, improvisations, and interpretations exist alongside the simultaneous and spontaneous. Basically, these are the main elements by which meaning is constructed in play, says Steinsholt.

Play's meaning, which the children in play create together (like people in carnival), is without results and remains unfinished and fragmented. What we have is the children's performance of actions, which create only part of the truth (Steinsholt, 1998).

From the outside, the playing children's carnivalesque lives may seem chaotic and incidental. However, there is a sense of a whole there, although it exists only as process, that is, as a process toward a *possible* whole. One could say that the whole, by the children involved in play, is glimpsed as a glowing dedication and an uninhibited unfolding through which they constantly make new relations and/or renew their relationships.

In the Center of Here-and-Now

As process, play creates an ongoing chain of new events and new stories, just as carnival does. The experience of a continually interesting here-and-now among the children involved, as illustrated by Bakhtin's carnival, defines when play is play and when it is not.

This brings me back to play's demanding alternation between tension and release and the aesthetical dramaturgy (see Kruse, 2016, in chapter 1). Normally, children in play cope with this alternation between levels, which are also known as the *telic level,* the goal-aiming producer's level, and the *para-telic level,* the level involving role-play wherein the children forget time and place and are intensively involved in play as an experience (Hellendoorn, 1994). The latter resembles the flow-experience (Csikszentmihalyi, 1990; see chapter 2). Typically, the carnival lifestyle creates such experiences (Steinsholt, 1998).

SUMMARIZING THE MAIN ASPECTS OF "MY" CARNIVAL

However, rather than talking about the symbols of the medieval carnival transferred to modern times and literature, as does Bakhtin, or talking about the "carnival lifestyle," as Steinsholt labels play, I will relate to music therapy improvisation as a "carnival place" with "carnival actions" (Stensæth, 2002, 2008). These labels are used to explore music therapy improvisation as a phenomenon that involves activities and doings that resemble the actions of the people participating in carnival. This is a basis for the responsiveness in music therapy improvisation. Summarized, the main carnival aspects are:

Music Therapy Improvisation as a "Carnival Place". Several music therapists have described music therapy improvisation as a "space" and "place" for interaction. Ansdell and Pavlicevic (2005) refer to "place" as a shared experience of the music's idiom, "with its connotations of laid-back jazziness, its characteristic body movements, its modes and textures of playing and singing" (p. 209). My use of "place" refers to music therapy improvisation as a metaphorical place created by the client and the music therapist as they attune to each other, the situation, and the world to make music and improvise. This place is *freedom-based*, possessing carnival's attraction, inspiration, and joyfulness. In short, it affords other types of unfolding compared to everyday activities; it becomes almost an escape from customary everyday activities.

As a Place Between the Real World and Carnival. Perhaps it is meaningful to say that music therapy improvisation creates a place *between* the "real" world and the world of carnival? This between-world is personal; it is created because of the client and therapist and their unique way of cultivating the music therapy improvisation. It is also different from many other forms of human interaction in that it *embraces* carnival actions such as the fragmented, irrational, processlike, insensible, comical, humorous, ridiculous, premeditative, improvisational, experimental, explorative, aesthetical, identifying, pretend, transcendental, virtual, and so forth.

Carnival Responses. The position that Bakhtin gives to response is salient in carnival. He in fact regards every utterance in carnival as a response. In this book's context, his view is taken perhaps even further. "Anything" that the client does—whether an instrumental sound or facial expression, whether acted out consciously or not—is treated as a responsive utterance. Therefore, "everything" that client and therapist do contains the potential to become material for their complex musical-relational dialogue.

Through the Carnival Spectacle. Carnival reveals how Jakob and Karla relate to the improvisation as a spectacle where they are free to go back and forth, move in and out, and try out new actions and ways of being together. The music serves as masks, allowing them to explore, play out, and take risks. They both seem to have a sense of "knowing" that they use the music as masks and that the "insensible" might occur. They also know that they can start over again if they want to, creating new themes and suggesting new directions for their interaction.

The Carnival-like Attraction. Its attraction and the carnival-like, freedom-based atmosphere inspire them and drag them into the place. In fact, they expect the music therapy improvisation to be a place of large engagement, one that might create the feeling of timelessness. Jakob and

Karla accept not knowing *where* to move on to; they just explore *how* to move on, while feeling free and safe to do so.

The Fragmentary Character. The musical-relational exploration is a way for Jakob and Karla to test out impulses and feelings and to play along with the more or less rational impulses they get. However, despite the fragmentary character of their actions, dialogicality is maintained: The struggle toward a whole is kept alive, by stepping out and making temporal finalizations (through musical cadences, for example) with great effort by the music therapist and by the music-making, which is always at hand.

Carnival as Improvisation. The carnival image recognizes the music therapy *as* improvisation. It moves the focus away from rule-based and strictly planned actions and toward spontaneous unfolding actions. Carnival actions are equivocal and surprising. Their strangeness creates tensions that exist on a threshold between Jakob and Karla and their musical-relational actions. It is this tension that keeps them going, that pushes them forward into new openness, new mysteries, making them want to go deeper and further. Sometimes it culminates in a joint attention, sometimes it does not, but as long they find the exploration magnetic, they keep going.

Carnival Ambivalence. We have seen that not knowing where to move to in their music, or what to do with it, easily creates ambivalence in Jakob and Karla. Yet there is little concern connected to this type of ambivalence, which is typical for carnival, too. It is the presence that is important, a presence that involves a continuous exchange and exploration of (new) musical ideas between them—rhythmically, melodically, or through contrasts. A section of The Guitar Excerpt presents that Jakob is totally interested, yet at the same time he is rather challenged and pushed by the music therapist:

> *(Jakob) crosses arms again but not as tightly as before, withdraws a little, crosses arms ... as if negotiating with himself ("Shall I let go—or shan't I?")* (see The Guitar Excerpt in chapter 4)

The utterance in the parentheses indicates that Jakob is both willing and unwilling at the same time. For a moment, the situation gets paradoxical: Jakob resists participating despite the fact that he is very interested and ready to act. He withdraws and moves out of the spectacle to hold himself for a second. Very soon he gets back into the spectacle again and starts playing along. This shows that acting on the carnival threshold engages him profoundly, so much so that it involves taking risks.

Risk-tempting Carnival. Risk-tempting in theories on music therapy improvisation is not a new discovery. Theories connected to the early interaction analogy have already ascertained this point. Music therapists Gro E. H. Tønsberg and Tonhild S. Hauge refer to Colwyn Trevarthen's theories when they suggest that music therapy improvisation involves "different psychological planes" and that one of the levels involves the risk-tempting testing of the sources of interaction (Trevarthen, in Tønsberg & Hauge, 2003, p. 7). The alternation between tension and release is recognizable, whether it is between entranced involvement and withdrawal, between surplus and opposition, and so on. My impression, however, is that carnival ambivalence is different; it is a riskier zone than the zone created between the mothers and the infants in early interaction. It is perhaps closer to the term "conflict," which Leontjev uses in his definition of play (see my presentation of play in chapter 2).

IS THE MUSIC THERAPIST A JESTER?

But how does the image of carnival fit with the role of the music therapist: Could she, for example, be the jester?

As we might know, initially, a jester was a professional clown employed to entertain a king or nobleman in the Middle Ages. The jester's role was to amuse them with jokes and to create a pleasurable atmosphere. Obviously, the music therapist's role could relate to that of a jester since she too must make sure that the atmosphere in the carnival-like music therapy improvisation is joyful and pleasurable.

Yet, her role includes more than this. She must above all make sure that the client feels safe in entering the carnival. This is part of her responsibility, which she must keep in mind while securing a joyful and pleasurable atmosphere. Her attention is therefore at two places simultaneously. We could perhaps say that the music therapist is "Janus-faced," because she must look in two directions at the same time.[20]

An intriguing question: How does the music therapist experience her double role as the responsible one and a jester in that particular part of The Guitar Excerpt where the client experiences carnival ambivalence? To grasp Karla's thoughts from within the live situation, it is interesting to return to what it is described in the logs immediately after The Guitar Excerpt:

Karla becomes aware of her own feelings, that it is time for her to move on, that it seems impossible for her to stay any longer within this intense mode and that she needs air—She needs to "breathe." Doesn't he need to "breathe," too ...?

Karla also becomes aware of her own pushing and thinks: "Is this too much for him?" "Can I go further?" She wonders if she is being too intervening, too "invading." Yet she senses that he is safe, that he knows what to expect, and she finds that it is time to open up and to offer him an instrument ... (see chapter 4)

The quotation shows that Karla intends to secure that Jakob feels safe as she listens attentively. It also shows that she is aware that the music therapy improvisation, which is in an "intense mode," moves on a carnival threshold. She senses that Jakob might feel insecure, even overly amused, and she is aware of her own actions and how they affect him. When she questions her own pushing, she even admits that she might cause the ambivalence that he experiences.

During carnival ambivalence, Karla questions her own role as a jester. Does she make it too amusing for him? She also questions whether she over- or underattunes Jakob's emotions. Like a responsible mother, she apprehends the dynamic forms of Jakob's actions and hence has a sense of his internal state. Yet, in contrast to being in the role of a mother, Karla is not so consolidating. Whereas the mother all-embraces the infant with her body and mind, Karla's focus is another. It is very much on Jakob's actions, whatever these might be. It seems as if Karla confronts Jakob's actions musically and thereby creates a way for her to enter the carnival spectacle together with him.

As we can see, the music therapist's role includes much more than just that of a jester. I therefore think that it is meaningful to call the music therapist a companion and an accompanist, as Ansdell and Pavlicevic (2005) proposed earlier (chapter 1). This means that she accompanies not only the client's actions in sound, but also the life of the client.

Inspired by Bakhtin, I would put it this way: Because she cannot play only for him, and because his engagement and interest require her personal commitment as well as her open-minded and authentic responses, she accompanies her own life, too.

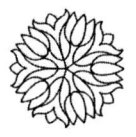

Chapter 13

MERGING PERSPECTIVES ON CARNIVAL, PLAYFULNESS, AND ACTION

This chapter merges the aspects of play with the aspects of carnival and action upon which I have elaborated in chapter 12. This chapter creates a premise for engaging in responsiveness in the music therapy improvisation. In this chapter, my ideas have more or less creatively taken over for Bakhtin's.

CONDITIONS FOR RESPONSIVENESS

A Playlike Condition

For responsiveness in music therapy improvisation to appear as a threshold phenomenon, playlike aspects are illustrative. Music therapy improvisation, like play and carnival, seems to work through the conflict between the two central components in human actions, that is, between the need to act and ways in which to perform the action. Yet, as we know, inspiration and contentment are also crucial here. Jakob's challenges to act versus his capability to act are also in play here.[21]

Whereas the need to act versus the challenges connected to ways in which to act relates to general and foundational psychology, as in Maslow's theory of self-actualization, the latter describes what it takes to provide inspiration and contentment, which is a presupposition for the individual to act freely and willingly (as in carnival).

Apparently, this is something that differs from person to person. Jakob has physical and mental handicaps and therefore needs help and preparation regarding this point. His action challenges are, for example, directly connected to the help he gets; in fact, his action challenges could be seen as a consequence of Karla's ability to incorporate his actions into a musical whole.

Thereafter, to create a tension, his action challenges must match, or even go against, his action capabilities, which in turn depend on his developmental age and aspects such as sensory apparatus and physical and mental capacity.

The tension between the Jakob's action capabilities and action challenges, which we know explains how to approach inspiration and contentment, also depends on the fact that he finds ways to act, too. Jakob will not act if he cannot feel a need to act, nor does he act if he cannot find a way to act. These are various aspects that create a playlike condition in the action performers that I will discuss in the following.

Carolyn Kenny on Play Conditions

Interestingly, in her book *The Field of Play*, Kenny discusses conditions as important considerations in music therapy (Kenny, 1995). From the study of theoretical roots, she finds four essential elements, which are (1) conditions, (2) fields of environments, (3) relationships, and (4) organization/self-organization. Out of these, at least if we are to consider music therapy improvisation as a process-oriented art and science, the least explored element is conditions. Kenny says (1995), "It is important to consider these 'conditions' even before the onset of the therapeutic relationship, since they may constitute nonverbal cues in the field" (p. 40).

I argue that for responsiveness to occur, music therapy improvisation requires the play condition within the client and the therapist. In the narrative, Jakob's as well as Karla's actions connect to tensions between such factors as intention, need, possibility, challenge, capability, opportunity, inspiration, and contentment. All of these aspects seem to predict each other. What is likely, and as I have tried to show, is that the intertwining of these enables music therapy improvisation to accommodate action.

The Presence of Several Levels of Consciousness

The various levels of consciousness could be present at the same time within the action performers. The action–intention relationship (cf. Figure 2) occurs on a phenomenological level and is not something that the client or the therapist thinks about in the music therapy improvisation. A client is normally not aware of such things as "action needs" either; instead, needs are realized as they are aroused and stimulated, for example, by the musical interaction.

For Jakob, the levels of consciousness are different from those of a client whose developmental age is higher. Because he acts mostly intuitively and impulsively, his actions seem to be performed without a high level of awareness. He does not worry about his "action capabilities." This, however, does not mean that his actions are constructed differently from those of a client who is more aware of what he/she is doing; rather, it means that his attention is different. Whereas other clients' attentions could be directed toward how to act—for example, how to play an instrument—Jakob's attention is more connected to the pleasure of acting.

For him, it probably does not really matter how the actions are performed. What does matter is to unfold and experience the actions as so interesting that he wants to continue. As for Karla, she acts both consciously and unconsciously; to accompany Jakob, she moves between various modes of consciousness. When she steps out of the improvisation, for example, she does not leave it; instead, she steps out to reflect-in-action (cf. Schön, 1983).

Practically, The Guitar Excerpt shows that Jakob's arm movements, next to solving his need to act with a way to act, are also a result of the tension created between his capabilities and challenges to act. To push his action capabilities and action challenges, Karla helps him. She performs her help actively and in musical terms. When he crosses his arms and withdraws, Karla pauses a little before she accompanies his dancing arms with flamenco-like playing on the guitar. By listening attentively to what he does, she tries to move "somewhere with him musically," as expressed in the narrative. She accompanies his dancing arms with flamenco-like playing on the guitar. When Jakob withdraws, she pauses, too. In this way, she shows him that she understands what he utters. She also shows that she trusts in the music to afford a way for her to create such understanding.

MATERIALIZING TIME ASPECTS IN THE IMPROVISATION BETWEEN JAKOB AND KARLA

One point that I believe is in sympathy with Bakhtin's world and is easily seen in the above presentation is that there is always dialectic between *chronos* and *kairos* (see Aldridge in chapter 1). The idea is to uphold tensions and not to become fully synchronized, a condition of which Figure 11 is a good illustration.

Figure 11. "Materializing" Time Aspects.

Nos. 7–8 in The Djembe Excerpt

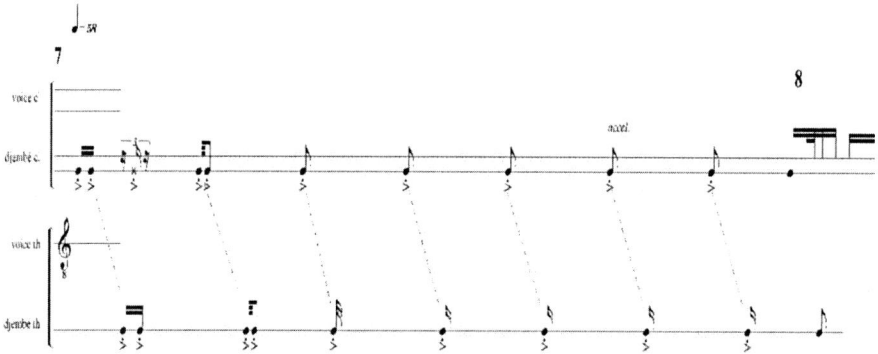

The dotted lines in the figure show that there is a delay between the responses of Jakob and Karla. These lines indicate that the asymmetry after a while establishes a regularity in their way of responding to each other.

Delayed Synchronicity or/and Participatory Discrepancies

What I am talking about here is not a question about "perfect timing," in the sense of being totally *synchronic* and doing the exact same thing at the exact same time. Trevarthen (1989) makes this point by saying that attunement is not all, just as a mother is seen not just to mirror, but also to extend her infant's proto-conversation by playfully and carefully judged *mis*-attunements. What we see is that for the players to become interested, there need to be variations or small discrepancies in the interaction, something that plays against a tight regularity, around the beat and out of tune.

Several music therapy thinkers agree on the importance of this aspect (Aigen, 2005; Aldridge, 2001; Ansdell & Pavlicevic, 2005; Ruud, 1998). Yet, to clarify how this could occur in the event, which is described as "delayed synchronicity" in my observation of the narrative with Jakob and Karla, it is necessary to question what causes the variation in the first place.

Evidently, the event involving the "delayed synchronicity" occurs as Jakob and/or Karla slightly displace the pulse in the juxtaposing beating on the djembe. The video recording of this place in the scores reveals that two aspects cause the pulse displacement. One is the fact that Jakob waits slightly longer than Karla before he hits the djembe with his hand. The fact that he leaves his arm and hand on the djembe when Karla beats the drum (as if he "listens" with his hand to what she does) seems to cause the delay. The other is that Karla exaggerates her beating by making large arm movements before she hits the djembe. Jakob needs time to feel her beat with his hand, and Karla needs time to perform her exaggerated and enlarged arm movements. This observation is described as if she makes some statement toward the client in the narrative (cf. chapter 4). An interesting aspect is that it is presumed in the narrative that the variation causes the dynamics and intensity in the music therapy improvisation to increase and that it brings in a feeling of tension, as if the interaction is fighting a complete synchronization (cf. chapter 4; Stensæth, 2008).

Having a "Real" Discussion on the Djembe?

Presumably, Jakob experiences the event as fascinating, or at least it seems as though this is the case from the way he focuses and concentrates on his playing. Something commented upon by several observers is that here he manages to stay within a pattern of doing the same thing over a longer period for the first time. Regarding Karla's experiences connected to this specific event, I will comment upon this by returning to the logs that describe this as follows:

> *She feels that they are having a "real" discussion: Jakob has his arguments and she has hers. Yet the discussion is without a transparent conclusion ...*

This quotation shows that the therapist, too, experiences the event with the delayed synchronicity as being intensively present, as if she is having a "real" discussion. One observer notices the intensity here and comments on the event by saying, "There is a serious quality to this work, to this 'being together' in the same space" (Stensæth, 2008, p. 126).

From what is known, there seems to be no doubt that the event is brought to the attention of both Jakob and Karla. Both are intently focused on each other and their playing, and the impression is therefore that at this stage of the improvisation they work hard, that they argue and negotiate.

Perhaps the event, because of the attention arousal caused by the delayed synchronicity, reveals a larger reciprocity in the interaction? If it does, this suggests that the ability *to time* becomes crucial. Eventually, responsiveness in music therapy improvisation is partly qualified by a sense of (good) timing among the participants and the music therapist in particular.

ACTION VERSUS INTERACTION

Interaction is an overriding theme in music therapy theories. From the therapist's perspective, the emphasis on interaction could be understood as a therapeutic consideration. Because the music therapist "wishes" that the client and the therapist would interact in the music therapy improvisation, she also finds this connection. Yet, to look for connections between the actions does not mean that the music therapist and the client share intentions, feelings, or internal emotional state. Many theories seem to create suitable models for the interpretations of such connections, but my point is that actions in music therapy improvisation are not always intended *as* interaction in the sense of being related to the person sitting opposite. They are also carnival actions, performed impulsively and intuitively within a collective setting. The players direct their actions toward the other's actions, but also toward themselves, the situation, and/or "the world," as Bakhtin could have put it. Their interaction is revealed as a continuous play with—and exploration of—actions and intentions. The effort also connects to the contemporizing and realizations of (many possible) actions and intentions.

Struggling with Actions and Each Other

Jakob and Karla's struggle is possible to exemplify when relating to the event in The Guitar Excerpt when Jakob starts to lift his arms: When he raises his arms in the air, he does so basically because he is stimulated by Karla's guitar-playing. Thereafter, it is Karla who reads his actions as an invitation for her to play the guitar as an accompaniment to his arm movements. Already there is a chain of actions going on in which there is a constant tension between intention and action (cf. Figure 2): Karla's intention to start him off realizes Jakob's actions (his arm movements). Then her guitar-playing realizes his intentions (to participate). Another explanation could be that his actions (his arm movements) realize her intentions (to develop the music and move somewhere with him musically). A process of diving into an *open future* emerges as they get entangled in the process:

> In this future, the potential of one's musical actions remains, in the very moment of the improvisation, unclear. But, as Bakhtin explains, such uncertainty is the precondition for pursuing freedom because one tries to constantly "other" oneself in order to maintain fluid identities. (Kanellopoulos, 2011a, p. 104)

No First Initiative

The event is paradoxical regarding the relationship between action and intention and which of them comes first and last. The chain of intentions and actions as well as the apparent "confusing" continuum makes this particular section powerful and intense.

In the observations, there were various opinions, even small contradictions, regarding which intentions or actions create the foreground, and it was not really possible to point out which comes first here, action or intention. The potential of their musical actions at this very moment of the improvisation remained unclear. At this point, the complexity connected to responsiveness as a dialogical process is brought to the forefront in an original version in music therapy improvisation: The initiative, as a first step in a chain of actions, does not exist; rather, it is erased and redefined, since an initiative is already a response. Thus, it is impossible to separate initiative from response in the music therapy improvisation. Every response points to the intertextuality of an utterance; it is always connected to other responses and cannot be separated from these either.

MAINTAINING A DIALOGICAL MIND-SET IN THE CARNIVAL

Naturally, because they are facing each other and approach the music-making willingly, Jakob and Karla will direct as well as synchronize their actions toward each other. Interaction, in the sense of sharing, could be seen as a consequence of their positioning and the inspiration they feel from the music-making. This suggests that music therapy improvisation affords a dialogical mind-set among those who take part in it. This mind-set posits that closure is not final, that there are always moments when something else could have happened. One of them could do something that escaped the other's attention. Karla, for reasons of which she was not aware within the moment, responded to Jakob's arm movements. She did not respond to his head movements or to the look in his eyes or to anything else that he did within the same moment. Jakob responded as he did for reasons that he did not take into account. Responsiveness involves such incidental choices, and for them to maintain dialogic, Jakob and Karla keep their music open, not closed or monologic.

Do Jakob and Karla show a dialogical mind-set in the narrative? Do the experienced music therapists, in their observations of the narrative, describe a dialogical "state of mind"? The answer is: They all do, although they use different words to describe it.

The Dialogical Mind-set, Seen from the Practical Level

On the practical level, which is within the setting where Jakob and Karla act, this is especially salient in the way they negotiate musically through their actions. If we stick to Bakhtin's linguistic terminology, their musical dialogue is similar to a verbal dialogue in which they would ask each other questions. Also, the descriptive observations and the analysis, which is from abstracted positions, reveal that music therapists ask questions, too: What is happening here? How do we/they precede? (Stensæth, 2008, pp. 126–136; see also the book's Prelude).

As we know from his descriptions of the response, Bakhtin would probably have said that a question holds an answer or that a question is already an answer. In my context, this suggests that music therapy improvisation involves not a fixed structure but a dialogical activity. In fact, to hold the answer, the question must already connect to the answer, as a tension.

Jakob Making Question Mark with his Arms

In the narrative, we have seen that Jakob, through his bodily utterances and expressions, asks questions within the live setting. An example of this relates to the section in The Guitar Excerpt when the client questions, "Shall I let go—or shan't I?"[22] Here he crosses his arms as an ambivalent action, just before he raises them, as in a dance. When he lets go of crossing his arms and raises them, it is as if he actually draws the question mark in the air. Apparently, Jakob does not direct his question toward Karla; instead, he directs it toward himself. Thus, the interaction occurs not primarily between him and the therapist; instead, it seems to be more like a self-dialogue (or what Bakhtin refers to as "inner dialogue").

Moreover, by asking, he seems to have already answered: When he crosses his arms in experiencing ambivalence, the questioning and the answering are so demanding that he moves out of the carnival spectacle. Yet, not to move back into the carnival spectacle, which I suppose is what he discusses with himself whether he should or should not do, is not an option. Therefore, his withdrawal from the spectacle, as well as his questioning, is paradoxical: Despite raising a question, he already has the answer.

Upholding the Dialogical Mind-set

As in carnival, this shows that the sequence of questions and answers is indifferent. Both are responses to the tension, either to a question or to an answer. The point seems to be to create enough tension to uphold the dialogical mind-set in them. A citation from the logs that refers to Karla's thinking connected to the phenomenological setting is a relevant illustration of the dialogical mind-set in her:

> *Karla gets the feeling that they are both apart and together at the same time. Is it Jakob who plays randomly with her, next to her, for him, for her? Does he feel that she plays with him, next to him, for herself, for him?* (see chapter 4)

We can tell from this citation that Karla asks herself questions about her actions in the music therapy improvisation and that she explores her understanding of them. The citation could also be an example of how many music therapists, when we think and act, create self-dialogues, just as I anticipated in the book's Prelude: "What does he feel? Why did I do what I just did? Was it important in any way? Why? For whom was it important?" And so forth.

Imagining the Other

Accepting the image of both Jakob and Karla "speaking" to each other with questions and answers acknowledges that there is a dialogue going on that is more than just an exchange of "words" and vocal sounds. By simultaneously observing and experiencing each other's actions and utterances, whether these are performed bodily or through vocal sounds, each of them relates to the other in a direct sense by looking "into the eyes of another" (as asserted by Bakhtin) in the music therapy improvisation.

Despite its short duration, an event from The Guitar Excerpt can illustrate some of the complexity connected to their way of "speaking together." Bakhtin's image of the Other is particularly relevant here. The example refers to an event when Jakob "moves his head a little to the side—away from the music therapist" and "keeps his eyes and mouth open … listens …." Because it is Karla who makes the music at this stage of the event, it is assumed that Jakob focuses his hearing to hear the music therapist better. His hearing and his interest are, in other words, interpreted as being directed toward the music therapist and her musical actions, as if he expects something to come from her.

Similarly, although not directly said in the observation, it is suggested that Karla acts as if Jakob expects something from her as she "changes groove while she sings 'restlessly' on a note (e) and plays rhythmically and distinctively (as ♪♪♪♪♪♪♪) on the AMaj7 chord" on the guitar.

Figure 12. Imagining the Other in The Guitar Excerpt.

Bars 7–12 in The Guitar Excerpt

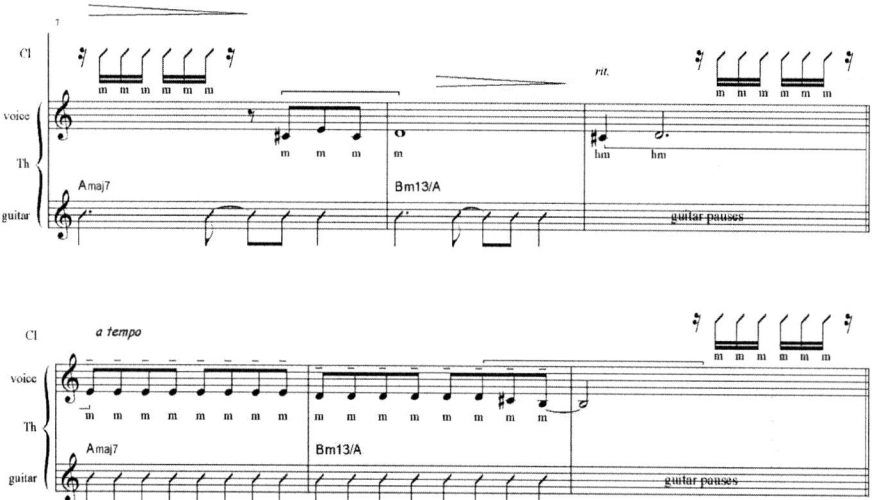

This part of their improvisation could indicate that Karla adopts her music to the vocal utterances of Jakob to "incorporate" his initiative. This could suggest that her attention is directed toward him and his response. Karla does not act just to avoid losing contact with him; rather, her attention and actions are directed toward the interaction as such, as a way of incorporating it into a larger musical whole. As we can see, this creates two dialogical connections: One is between Jakob and Karla, and the other is between their relationship and the music-making. Prime dialogical connections here are therefore the client, the therapist, and their musical relation.

Karla Exploring Ventriloquism

One place in the observation that follows from The Guitar Excerpt as shown above is especially interesting and illustrates the complexity. This is when the narrative (chapter 4) suggests that Jakob hears his own voice performed by the voice of Karla, as if he thinks, "Doesn't her music sound 'familiar'? Do I hear [or am I imagining] that she is imitating me and my voice and my way of singing?" The event suggests that Karla, the music therapist, just like a ventriloquist, "speaks" with the voice of the client and that she does so in order for him to hear his own voice and thereby become aware of his Self. In other words, Jakob experiences himself through Karla's voice, which she performs as an imitation of him. Yet, he does not experience just an imitation of his own voice; instead, he experiences a *realization* of his own voice.

This suggests that it is not just Karla's imitation skills that are important here; instead, it is her ability to empathize with Jakob. She lends herself to the process, and, like a ventriloquist, she gives voice to the doll that speaks with the voice of Jakob, while simultaneously being the therapist. Possessing the role of the ventriloquist who observes the whole scene, she offers Jakob a response that is unlike other responses.

Really, this event shows how the music therapist makes the client's consciousness "audible": She acts him out loud, so to speak. Moreover, this process reveals another dialogical connection, one between the client and the doll, in which the music therapist represents the client.

Normally, the latter type of dialogue occurs within a person, for example, between an old and a new "I" within a person. However, here the internal dialogue has become external with the help of the music therapist. In a therapy context, this is an important point, especially if the client is not able to experience himself in this way without the help of the therapist.

As it is transcribed into a music therapy improvisation, the complexity of this event shows a pragmatic incorporation of other consciousnesses in the music therapy improvisation, indicating a polyphonic state of mind in the therapist. Apparently, as a music therapist, although very much focused on Jakob, Karla continuously thinks of the therapeutic outcome and his well-being. Therefore, in the back of her head, she pays attention to others' consciousnesses as well, especially those of his parents and his caretaker (who sits next to him). Eventually, responsiveness in music therapy improvisation, such as in the case of Jakob and Karla, succeeds in keeping several consciousnesses in play—independent of who "speaks."

SUMMING UP

Bakhtin's carnival is a good metaphor for how the figures based in the action–intention relationship connect to a live situation (cf. Figure 2). In the zone between carnival and reality, and through the carnival actions, their tension, and their release, Jakob can unfold freely. Whatever he does will be accepted and dealt with. Even ambivalent and risk-tempting actions are welcome. The unburdening carnival unfolding leads Jakob to experience regeneration and revitalization from his participation.

However, what this perspective primarily shows is a premise for any therapy: An individual's desire to do (action) something (activities) meaningful (intentional) together (intersubjective and interpersonal) requires a shareable situation, one that is accessible to two (or more) players' consciousnesses at the same time.

Bakhtin's ideas show the need for the music therapist to welcome uncertainty, tensions, and conflicts. For a client like Jakob, as long as he feels safe and free, ambivalence and resistance could be seen as signs of "health." They reveal that he is able to get involved while still holding Self. As his music therapist, Karla is responsible for taking his process in a healthy direction. Her role is to support him in the exploration of his boundaries.

Because Jakob's body language is his first language, he expresses his exploration and whatever he experiences from it through his body, whether through arm movements, facial gestures, vocalization, and so on. One could say that externally his actions pave an internal path through which he, with help from Karla, can understand himself better.

This process of going in and out of (the spectacle) and backward and forward (on the action–intention axis) reveals that responsiveness in music therapy improvisation includes a range of actions, among which are those of a less rational type and those which I have called carnival actions. Some actions are immediately experienced as meaningful within the context, while in others the meaning emerges as process. Some actions imply carnivalesque exploration; through these—and by using the music as masks—the client and the therapist can pretend, seek, and try out transcendent experiences.

This shows again how the action–intention relationship is a boundary phenomenon. An action does not proceed just between a client and a music therapist; it also exists between action and intention, between synchronization and discrepancies, between content and outcome, between paradoxes and rationality, and so forth. Even the action's meaning is dynamic.

I argue that music therapy improvisation moves in the tension offered by these between-spaces and that it is the experience of time within the context of the live setting that decides what meaning is present. One could say that the label "actions of musical-relational synchronization" that derived from the narrative reveals that actions must be experienced as meaning-*full* to become kairotic. Their meaning is, as Bakhtin would point out, entirely based in the chronotope of every situation.

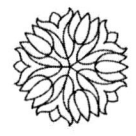

Chapter 14

"Musical Answerability:" A Theory on Responsiveness in Music Therapy Improvisation Inspired by Bakhtin

With meaning, I give answers to questions.
Anything that does not answer a question is devoid of sense for us.
—Mikhail Bakhtin—

The process that started my work with the present book emerged as an intuitive feeling of exploring existential topics when I have been making music with other people. This feeling has been even more prominent in me as a music therapist when I have been improvising with a client. I now see my intuition as a line of thought that has pervaded my whole life, both personally and professionally, from my time as a student at the École d'Humanité to my practice as a music therapist, to my role as a researcher in music therapy.

In my "new" image, responsiveness is emphasized as freedom of expression. It is an invention that is accompanied by a particular sense of responsibility which is intersubjective and secures openness, fights finalizations, and puts our musical actions into dialogue with others. Freedom, in this sense, is not a particular state of being; "it is a condition continually sought after" (cf. Kanellopoulos, 2011b, p. 125). It is also that which attracts us all, as well as client and therapist, to the musical improvisation and makes us want to act and take part in it. This is a premise.

Introducing my Theory

With inspiration from Bakhtin, I have articulated a theory that is a way of thinking about responsiveness in music therapy improvisation. I will label my theory *musical answerability*. I have already suggested two levels of reflection as significant in this regard (cf. Lillis, 2003): One is responsiveness as given, and to the "nature" of improvisation as an intuitive way of exploring and creative being in the here-and-now. The other level is responsiveness as a dialogical ideal, as something that is challenging and not always possible to sustain over time but important and meaningful to struggle for.

I want to underline that my transposing of insights of Bakhtin's world into a theory is not a finalized project. It belongs to an ongoing chain of unfinalized music therapy dialogues. One voice is never enough—it takes at least two to become life (cf. Bakhtin, 1994). Similarly, in music therapy ...

> the work is never complete or finished and never entirely in and of itself; but only insofar as it provides a commentary on what has gone before and offers a vehicle to consider novel extensions and additional resources in response to new contexts. (White & Peters, 2011, p. 8)

Every music therapy improvisation and its individuals create in the same way unique events that engage new sets of voices, which are connected to past as well as future improvisations.

To characterize how human dialogue involves several voices, we have learned that Bakhtin borrows the term "polyphony" from the world of music. I suggest "taking it back" by transferring his understanding of it to my focus in this book. The process of ventriloquism, as it has been creatively manifested before, exposes how complex the voice issue can be. It shows, theoretically speaking, how other voices are present in our process of understanding other people and the world around us. Music therapy discourses, to resist finalized monologism wherein one theory becomes the current "truth," therefore involve open-ended dialogues.

My theory on musical answerability is a contribution to this process. Its dialogical, ethical, and aesthetical aspects are prominent, and I will sum these up as follows.

Musical Answerability as a Dialogical Theory

Musical answerability is a dialogical theory on the meaning-making process in music therapy improvisation. It locates meaning in the dialogical relationship between client and therapist, which raises genuine, serious, interested questions. This refers to Bakhtin, who says,

> With meaning, I give answers to questions. Anything that does not answer a question is devoid of sense for us. Meaning always responds to particular questions. Anything that does not respond to something seems meaningless to us; it is removed from dialogue. (Bakhtin, 1986b, p. 145)

Transferred to music therapy improvisation, this means that each player does not know the answer to each question he/she asks and that the other player takes each question seriously and replies to it to the best of his or her knowledge (Matusov, 2015).

As a dialogical theory, musical answerability refers to responsiveness in music therapy improvisation as communication, culture, and action:

- *As communication*, it resonates with life itself. "To be means to communicate," Bakhtin said (1984, p. 287). This part connects my theory to Bakhtin's existential worldview.
- *As culture*, it is a radical and anti-authoritative communication event, one that represents a way of creating and cultivating local, democratic microcultures. Bakhtin's carnival is a suited metaphor for how this works.
- *As action*, it is a creative musical and relational exploration between players who co-author their doings while actively approaching each other as unfinalized strangers. As strangers, they are constantly in the process of realizing themselves and are resistant to any finalizing definition or end point of an understanding of each other. Their musical playing therefore involves surprises and unexpected actions, which makes the element of improvisation open to responsiveness.

Musical Answerability as a Theory of Ethics

Musical answerability is a theory of ethics, too. Here, responsiveness becomes a deed, as an ethical obligation to engage lovingly and artistically in answerable acts with people around us, perhaps especially with people who are in need. With engagement and interest, personal commitment, and open-minded and authentic responses, the therapist accompanies the client's life and being in the here-and-now. Through a mode of consciousness and through her intersubjective relation to the Other and the world, she relates to the music therapy improvisation as artwork that forms her identity, too, not just the client's. The latter aspect creates a link to the aesthetics in musical answerability.

Musical Answerability as a Theory of Aesthetics

Musical answerability is also a theory of aesthetics. Authoring responsiveness aesthetically in the practical situation requires that the therapist involve herself aesthetically in their musical-relational interaction. Karla must engage genuinely in Jakob, face-to-face, with a "willingness to be more lover than beloved" (cf. Emerson, 2000, p. 284). She needs to show that she loves "life from without, in the place where it is not for itself, where it is turned outside itself and is in need of an outside activity beyond meaning" (Bakhtin, 1984, p. 175). By stepping outside of the improvisation (without leaving it) every once in a while, she makes temporal finalizations perceiving what escaped the immediacy of the event (cf. Kanellopoulos, 2011b). Her outsideness refers to the act of transcendence, whereby contents of lived experiences are placed on "a new plane of existence" (Bakhtin, 1984, p. 18), in the work of art.

In the narrative of Jakob and Karla, the music therapist got images of Michelangelo's *Creation of Adam* in her mind during the music therapy improvisation. This painting, she felt, resembled her feeling of how she and Jakob in their improvisation reached out to each other, that they *almost* touched, but that she at the same time actually experienced stepping outside the course of action for a moment and seeing the client and herself in the music therapy improvisation from another level (from what I called the "roof perspective").

This is an example of how the music therapist might move between levels of consciousness in order to respond to various voices while she intuitively searches for (aesthetical) wholeness. Bakhtin thinks that because we always struggle for wholeness in our lives, we make temporary finalizations like this. This is characteristic of the aesthetic act. It is also essential for the act of understanding and for our very possibility of perceiving the distinctiveness and wholeness of particular acts (cf. Kanellopoulos, 2011b).

Placing Musical Answerability within Three Perspectives

I will cover three perspectives within musical answerability: the existential, the sociological, and the practical-relational.

Musical Answerability, an Existential Perspective

Glimpsing an existential perspective, à la Bakhtin, musical answerability suggests that the client and music therapist in music therapy improvisation do not share only actions or music; they also share existence as an event. In this sense, musical answerability connects to the existential project; it is understood as a human condition, without which we cannot exist. For the client and his being, the therapist's obligation could be crucial. For his voice to be heard, he depends on her to treat his utterances (verbal or performed bodily) as dialogical activity and as existential utterances.

Interestingly, the word "exist" comes from the Latin word *exsistere*, which means "to come forth, be manifest."[24] For the client, this could suggest that the improvisation is especially meaningful in the sense that it creates a chance for him/her to come forth. The most obvious way for Jakob to manifest himself is to move his body, which he does easily with inspiration from music. In other words, his characteristic arm movements have a meaning that goes beyond the ability to move a limb. Perhaps one could say that when he raises his arms, it is a metaphor for him reaching out for the world, for existence?

Musical Answerability, a Social Perspective

To unify with Bakhtin's world, musical answerability is above all a social project. It is about externalizing and internalizing and about how to become part of a larger community. Interestingly, and as many music therapists know, the terms "community" and "communication" come from the Latin word *communicare*, which means "to impart, share" or "to make common."[25] Musical answerability, then, is about experience-sharing by making common effort, that is, through "actions of musical-relational synchronizing" (cf. Stensæth, 2008). Isolation is its contrast. Hence, musical answerability at this level is in a way also about avoiding isolation.

If we use Jakob's arm movements as an image again, this suggests that by moving and raising his arms, Jakob reaches out for *someone*. This need not be the one to whom Jakob feels closest, such as his mother, for example. Instead, it could be anyone who is willing to face him, actively and authentically. I suggest that musical answerability, to borrow the words of Ansdell and Pavlicevic (2005), "holds together" the mutually constructed speaking, moving, and "'being with' of persons in a social world" (p. 200).

Ruud suggests music therapy improvisation to be a phenomenon with a miniature social system (Ruud, 1998). This view suggests that actions as communication are socially dependent. The improvisation becomes a live experience of mutual tuning-in through time.

The observers of the narrative share the impression that the musical announcements made by Jakob and Karla are not isolated utterances but attempts at creating a whole. It is not easy to tell from the sound who plays what in the improvisation between them. Paradoxically, then, the observers see that the turn-taking is no longer turn-taking but two persons playing as one, as a We. Responsiveness, on this level, far from being static, is a living, social phenomenon. Musical answerability dynamically contributes the meanings that can be made.

Yet, in the course of the improvisation, it is difficult—impossible, perhaps—to tell who affects whom or what affects what. What their responses mean depends on their particular *addressivity:* who is being addressed and what is being addressed. For Jakob and Karla, this suggests that their musical actions do not exist in isolation. Instead, they belong to a chain of communication. Therefore, action is a vital theme here, too, a cantus firmus, so to speak. The action's sociality defines its meaning.

Musical Answerability, a Practical-Relational Perspective

Musical answerability is *situated*. This means that Jakob's arm movements can be dialogized within a practical context.

Together with Per Lorentzen (2001), the psychologist, I suggest that Bakhtin's dialogical perspective in a therapy situation implies a *practical-relational understanding* (Lorentzen, 2001). This view suggests that the music therapist must not just meet the client as he is (cf. Nordoff & Robbins, 1977) and does not necessarily present a normalized picture of how he *should* be; it means approaching the situation and the client with willingness and trust so that their actions can unfold freely.

Musical answerability shows that a client and a therapist becoming musically answerable depends on music and actions within the setting. The primary task at this level is to bring the improvisation close, to contemporize, even to ridicule and laugh, like people do in carnival. In this perspective—and to play with words again—improvisation becomes a way to *improve a situation* (Stensæth, 2008).

On this level, musical answerability comprises the practices of the required "closeness ethics" and/or "situational ethics" (cf. Martinsen, 2003, 2005; see chapter 1). Only in this way can the music therapy improvisation become a dialogical alternative where "actions about" at some level are always "actions between" and where "actions between" include all possible dialogical connections between the client and the therapist, their relationship, and the music.

A practical-relational understanding includes a body-based perspective.[26] As suggested in chapter 1, the body experiences meaning, too. Hence meaning is not an entirely intellectual process; rather, meaning involves both body and mind. When Jakob raises his arms into the air, his body responds before his mind. This is typical for Jakob, because he is without words and experiments first with meaning through bodily actions.

Yet, as an exemplar of many settings where actions create the foreground, this perspective is essential in music therapy improvisation in general, too. Very often, in any improvisation, the players act with their bodies before they reflect. They act first, but not necessarily without intention or direction. Trondalen (2016) describes this as follows: "The human body is a carrier of subjectivity that recognizes the other as a body subject, the significance of bodily phenomena being in the forefront" (p. 33).

A consequence of a practical-relational understanding is that the music therapy improvisation develops in such a way that it becomes personal for both the client and the therapist; the improvisation turns into a shared interpersonal "property," a community, as We. After some time, they develop a common personal history, from which their future actions develop as themes between them (cf. Holck, 2004).

Music, with its parameters of rhythm, melody, harmony, timbre, and so forth, simply offers the most obvious possibilities for creating the required tensions through which the improvisation receives direction and aim. The music helps them both in becoming answerable. The clue here, which is also a paradox, is that because it is so easy to create order and meaning, music allows much chaos.

Yet, by integrating carnival's paradoxical mix of chaos and order, reality and unreality, and possibility to vary and to uphold an interesting here-and-now, the impression given is that there is still a sense of whole. One could say that due to the way in which music therapy improvisation is cultivated (indigenously), musical answerability emerges as an obvious option through which the client can unite the lived experiences of the musical actions in himself and the unity of his answerability. In this sense, responsiveness in music therapy improvisation involves a pragmatic solution of how to act together and be "in the process of."

SUMMARIZING THE MAIN CHARACTERISTICS OF THE THEORY

The following sections summarize the main aspects of my theory. Musical answerability is brought forth:

By Keeping Differences in Play. Musical answerability is most of all an adequate form to verbally express how I understand responsiveness in music therapy improvisation as authentic human life and an open-ended dialogue. It is a process that involves dialogicality, which means accepting that every music therapy improvisation is paradoxical, that it includes familiarity *and* strangeness. Musical answerability emphasizes, in fact, the need to keep differences in play in its process and goal. This is another premise behind responsiveness.

With a Dialogical Basis. Bakhtin's dialogue is considered a key issue as a process of meaning-making, permeating "all relationships and manifestations of human life in general, everything that has meaning and significance" (Bakhtin, 1984, p. 40). This image refers to a grand conception of his dialogue. In such an image, musical answerability is an aesthetical and ethical engagement with oneself, the Other, existence, and the world. It is a living genre of communication and involves intentional acts of intersubjectivity and alterity.

Through the Personal and Quaint Response. The idea with responsiveness in music therapy improvisation is that a response, coming from both client and therapist, because it holds the intention to share and understand, is always personal and quaint. The client and the therapist are different individuals who occupy different positions in the world. Neither of them can occupy the other's or another's place (without losing their own). Each of them is an individual with a different personality, and the goal is never to mirror perfectly or to become identical with the other.

With Inspiration from Aspects of Creative Music Therapy. Musical answerability refers to a specific culture of improvisation in music therapy, which in my case relates to the Nordoff and Robbins tradition. This tradition is a dense and open musical improvisation that involves evoking musical responses, developing musical skills, and interresponsiveness. My theory does not share Nordoff and Robbins's view on the music child, as an inborn capacity in the client. Instead, it is based in Bakhtin's idea that "truth is not born nor is it be found inside the head of an individual person, it is born *between people* collectively searching for truth" (Bakhtin, 1984, p. 110). Responsiveness in this perspective becomes *inter*individual and intersubjective: "The idea is a living event which is played out where two consciousnesses meet dialogically" (Bakhtin, 1984, p. 72). Musical answerability requires, therefore, both client and therapist to actively explore each other to become musically answerable to the improvisation, each other, and the world.

Through Actions of Musical-Relational Synchronizing. My illustration of action as a phenomenon reveals how musical answerability is activated in the players. It shows how Karla and Jakob spontaneously explore and balance intentions and actions in their improvisation. I have characterized the process as "actions of musical-relational synchronizing." The label displays how they struggle to synchronize their actions and to find connections in their doings: When Jakob moves his arms characteristically, his initiation is understood as an initiation that may transcend Karla's initiation, while her evaluation of his response may transcend his response, and so on (cf. Matusov, 2015).

With Musical Dramaturgy. Musical answerability shows that because music is so inspiring and because it allows many variations of structure and dynamics, it is very appropriate as the creative and aesthetic form with which the players can create a dramaturgy of their improvisation. As I have implied before, Bakhtin's emphasis of dissonances and discrepancies is especially inspiring, not just because these parameters are directly recognizable in musical terms, but also because these characteristics are often left out in music therapy theories' continuing search for agreement, consensus, harmony, and well-being.

Through the Carnival-like Status. The improvisation's carnival-like status promotes actions that are freedom-based, fragmentary, chaotic and paradoxical, even ridiculous and ironic, but also fulfilling and pleasant. Its irresistible driving force engages Jakob and Karla to act in a way such that they almost feel that they cannot do it differently.

Through the Balancing of Tensions. The little word "between" is significant. It uncovers the crucial aspect of balancing, that to uphold an interesting here-and-now among the participants requires a balancing *between* tensions; between tension and release, the tension stretches between reality and fiction, overattune and underattune, challenging and too challenging, structure and chaos, rational and irrational, whole and part, and so forth. However, the most evidential tension, at least if the idea is to maintain an improvisational character, is that between action and intention. This tension, which relates directly to the play condition, is needed to allow meaning to emerge within the process.

With Magnetic Attraction. Typically, as the narrative of Jakob and Karla shows, the music therapy improvisation involves resistance and confusion just as much as harmony and synchronization. This is required to establish tensions and motivation to push the improvisation forward and create new interest in the players. Its strong, magnetic attraction and feeling of presence cause a carnival-like absorbing interest, sometimes so intensively that it almost feels *too* stimulating.

With Room for Ambivalent Feelings. Feeling ambivalent and not knowing what to do might be the result. Both players can solve the challenge by making temporal finalizations, for example, by stepping out of the spectacle (without leaving it) before stepping in again. The improvisation's carnivalesque character will inform them that they are free to do so. Risk-tempting actions are welcome, because the musical-relational framing holds the players and makes them feel safe.

Through the Musical-Relational "Ought." The mix of modes and creative exploration explains why the musical-relational "ought" is activated in Jakob and Karla in their improvisation. It derives from the musical encounter between client and therapist, who approach each other actively in the musical improvisation. In this view, their relationship is in itself part of their musical improvisation. The "ought" emerges from the improvisation when the players feel obligated to respond and act upon the Other in a musical-relational way. It also involves an expectation of being surprised and encountering strangeness (the Alter) and of experiencing the improvisation as that of being individual, unique, and unrepeatable.

Through a Community of Music Therapy Improvisation. Both client and therapist are needed to co-author their actions so that they can become impacted by traces from both of them. Their improvisation gets an identity as "theirs"; it creates the feeling of the We, a Community, where their "here-and-now"–centered agency allows improvisation, differences, creativity, struggle, originality, diversity, and uniqueness. Transposed to the narrative, this suggests that with Jakob and Karla, in every situation, in every improvisation they co-author together, Karla is expert in her tandem efforts with Jakob.

Through Experiences of Sharing (not Doing the Same Thing). Jakob and Karla might experience the feeling of sharing, but they (probably) do not experience the same thing. The process *toward* synchronization is emphasized, since doing the exact same thing at the exact same time is not interesting, especially not in the long run. An aspect such as participatory discrepancies is essential.

Through Co-Authorship. The therapist's self is answerable *for* the authorship of her responses. To qualify co-authorship of the responsiveness, she doubts her own voices to allow the client's voices to influence hers. To do so, she "others" herself and willingly reads his strange utterances as potential statements. For Jakob, who is a client without words, Karla might read his movements and/or bodily utterances as external evidences of his internal experiences.

With a Dialogical Mind-set. Karla's role is different from Jakob's. To feel the personal obligation to respond without losing her professional obligation requires a dialogical mind-set in her. This presupposes that she tries out the role of being the Other for Jakob and leaves space for him while also doubting her own voice (e.g., theories, prejudices, what she knows, etc.). It also assumes that she is a close other for Jakob, one who is personally willing and professionally able to read his needs and desires while transferring them to musical negotiation material from moment to moment in the course of the improvisation.

By Being a Participant in the Other's life. The music therapist's positioning of herself as a participant and not just a spectator in Jakob's life is desirable. Karla can achieve the required authenticity when she takes into account not only her own emotions of the other-in-the-self and the actual other, but also an attention to the improvisation as a process that is connected to her life (cf. White & Peters, 2011). Her "answerable act" is then offered as an ontological feature of her as a subject. It is an act and a deed that is constitutive of Being. Therefore, she cannot see the client as solely an object for therapy. She cannot view the improvisation as something delivered from her to the client either. No, musical answerability, with its Bakhtinian inspiration, rejects any quick-fix demonstrations of music therapy improvisation as solely a technique or a model.

By Looking for Meaning Outside (and Between) the Players. Evidently, musical answerability suggests that meaning is not found entirely inside the heads of the client and the music therapist; rather, it is created between them, through actions and between their actions. Musical answerability is a discourse in which the action performers can describe and redescribe, agree and dispute, construct and contest their actions musically. It holds that there is not such a thing as *one* meaning or *one* response, **one** answer. Instead, the process of finding meaning is played out between them.

Through a Polyphony of Meanings. The theory reveals that there is an orchestral polyphony of possible meanings and answers involved in music therapy improvisation. In the sense that they interconnect, all meanings involved have the potential to condition others. They are heteroglot, as Bakhtin would have put it. To get hold of his/her unity of answerability, the client and the therapist explore the meanings actively and authentically, but also with joy and seriousness.

With an Ethical Uniqueness. Every musical utterance within the improvisation therefore acquires its uniqueness from the player's unique obligation to follow a particular pathway and is not the simple result of abiding by the rules of a particular "logic." From a Bakhtinian point of view, this is an ethical uniqueness (cf. Kanellopoulos, 2011b).

Through Chronotope. Musical answerability is chronotope; it is bound to time and space. It has an intrinsic connectedness that refers to its specific situation that makes up its own concrete whole. The meaning of it cannot be separated from its context. Jakob and Karla's improvisation is responsive only to *its* situation, to *those* people who are in it, and to *their* process and *their* moment of time (cf. Keunen, 2011; White & Peters, 2011).

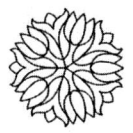

Chapter 15

DISCUSSING THEORY ASPECTS

Has my fascination for Bakhtin and his dialogue turned my theory in a monological direction, as if musical answerability is the one and only possible perspective on responsiveness in music therapy improvisation? Any attempt to be authoritative in my idea of music answerability would be misguiding. My theorizing is not an attempt to constrain, purify, or force my comprehension onto you, the readers. That would make my ideas monologist, monovoiced, even dead. Instead, my comprehension involves the creativity of transcending music therapy improvisation as something already given—given cultural norms, knowledge, practice, skills, attitudes, and so on.

In its own turn, the transcendence involves uncertainty and risk. Comprehension is always risky, just as entering any hermeneutic universe is risky (cf. Matusov, 2015). Understandings, preunderstandings, and interpretations are polyphone and heteroglot, connecting to other areas, ideas, and theories. This is a dialogical process. So, when we together, when you, the readers, and I engage in the comprehension process, it becomes dialogical. For this to become authoritative depends upon the book's mutual interest in us (i.e., interaddressivity) (Matusov, 2015).

Bakhtin's ideas operate on many levels and through many perspectives, but they are most of all a meta-theoretical view on human (musical) interaction. His perspectives, as metaphors, inspire my thinking of micro-settings as well, such as the one with Jakob and Karla. With new glasses, we might see more clearly how one part could create a new whole or vice versa.

I will discuss the challenges connected to my theoretical operation in the following.

MUSICAL ANSWERABILITY AS AN INTERLEVEL THEORY

The term "interlevel theory" means "between levels." The need for the term "interlevel theory" could be described as follows:

> The main point of the use of the term "interlevel" is to draw attention to the use of different entities at different levels of aggregation functioning in the same theory (or model) (Schaffner, in Kvernbekk, 2005, p. 88).

Kvernbekk (2005), the education theorist, explains the relation between the levels as a part–whole relation. To illustrate this, she explains that a magnitude s2 may be on a higher aggregation level than s1 if s1 is part of s2. The qualities connected to s2 are not just the sum of its parts; instead, it is better to say that the whole has a quality that differs from the sum of the parts. Yet, because the whole is sometimes problematic to define exactly and delimit, a more flexible view of it is required.

From my perspective, although it is rather technical, Kvernbekk's illustration is meaningful. First, it explains how Jakob's arm movement (s1), which is an action within the live setting that is understood as an utterance and part of the dialogue between him and Karla, could also connect to a larger whole, which I have called a unity of a musical answerability (s2). My theory on musical answerability in this way creates a return to my preunderstanding, where I view music therapy improvisation as part of an ecological system. This perspective could suggest that Jakob's arm movements have an ecological overtone.

Interestingly, Bateson's (1972) concept of context, in which action and utterance create the point of departure, seems to be a fruitful comment on this perspective:

> I speak of action or utterance as occurring "in" a context, and this conventional way of talking suggests that the particular action is a "dependent" variable, while the context is the "independent" variable. But this view of how action is related to its context is likely to distract the reader—as it has distracted me—from perceiving that ecology of the ideas which together constitute the small subsystem which I call "context." ... It is important to see that particular utterance or action as *part* of the ecological subsystem called context and

not as a product or effect of what remains of the context after the piece we want to explain has been cut from it. (p. 338)

This perspective suggests that an action and an event, such as that of Jakob's arm movements, influence the construction of the context and the whole. Its parts, which need not be "inside" the whole, put the whole together. Pragmatically understood, this means that Jakob's arm movements, which could be a general expression of his enthusiasm and therefore occur also in other settings, construct the whole when they are understood as ecology and part of a unifying theory.

It would be meaningful to place my theory about musical answerability within a sociological perspective. This suggests that the unifying (or general) theory could be socialization. With inspiration from Bakhtin's sociological perspectives, I see that I have acquired a more adequate framework for understanding intricate relations, such as those between theory and practice or even between action and intention. In this process, the main task has been to connect my thought constructions to the sociological perspectives, which I have internalized from both the empirical and the theoretical elaborations, and my understanding of Bakhtin's perspectives.

According to Kvernbekk, a meta-theoretical perspective like this allows the incorporation of situational appraisals and personal judgments on the part of the practitioner into the application of a given theory. My understanding of the event with Jakob's arm movements is an example of this: Through the reflexive maneuvers between the empirical material and the theoretical discussions of them, it has been possible to argue that Jakob's actions provide a picture of what my theory is. As Kvernbekk suggests, it is the different levels of abstraction that qualify a theory such as the present one as semantically oriented.

IS THE THEORY MUSIC-CENTERED?

I do find it problematic to center my theory. Although music is a vital source, my theory is not necessarily music-centered. An illustration that could be interesting in this respect refers to the logs, where I speak with the voice of Karla, as the music therapist from within the setting:

> *Karla "sees" Jakob: all of him. She sees the slim body in the wheelchair, his face with this expectant, interrogative, and slightly frightened look, his arms moving in all directions, and*

how he suddenly crosses them every once in a while, and she sees the center of his body making small shaking movements. She remembers how she perceives his sounds and his body as one expression, an expression that is somewhat chaotic, but full of spirit—always ready to move somewhere musically, always ready for the next step! A question (which she remembers has come to her before) emerges: Is this his surplus of energy and action that cries to come out?

As we can see, I do not music-center my thinking while reflecting-in-action. Typically, my impulses emerge as sensations, of which the musical experience of him is one part. Yet, to connect to a unifying theory, I do see that playing music with others could be a microcosm of the challenge put to all human beings to achieve personal satisfaction within social structures.

As we have seen throughout the book, there seem to be many aspects involved with responsiveness in music therapy improvisation. It becomes difficult to focus solely on one of them. Music is one aspect, and as we know by now, in my understanding, action is a primary aspect, too. The same goes for relationship. All of these aspects, and the way they interrelate, create some kind of a center of my thinking.

RETURNING TO THE QUESTION OF AUTHORSHIP

This book and its theory have shed light on the challenges connected to the music therapist's understanding and interpretation of process and result. It shows that there are so many potential voices involved in her understanding. Through his use of heteroglossia, Bakhtin reminds us that we must be aware of the authoritative discourses.

Dialogism, says Holquist (1981), is the characteristic epistemological mode of a world dominated by heteroglossia. All utterances are heteroglot, meaning that at any given time, in any given place, they belong to a set of conditions—whether social, historical, or physiological—which ensure that a word uttered in a particular place at a particular time will have a meaning different from what it would have under any other conditions (Bakhtin, 1981, 1984). Where does this leave me in my theory-building?

In Norway, as I have said before, we often claim to have a humanistic perspective on music therapy. I have also placed myself within this perspective. To author my interpretation of responsiveness in music therapy improvisation, I have asked myself: What discourses in the humanistic perspective are authoritative in my thinking, and have these surpassed others? Have I, for example, as a humanistically oriented music therapist, been constantly looking for harmony and positive results and at the same time overlooking misunderstandings or other aspects that also may influence the meaning-making?

To avoid the influence of dominant theoretical perspectives, I have tried to set aside what I know and instead listen openly and carefully to what the world might have taught me in every moment of action. I have learned that while I am in it, it is the moment (and everyone and everything present) that creates the foreground and tells me what to do and how to proceed, not the humanistic music therapy. I have also learned that it is difficult, even impossible, to bracket out my preunderstanding in a way that I am completely open and unbiased to the impulses I get. This is not what Bakhtin wants either, so here, too, the point with authorship is collaboration and authentic involvement with co-authors.

Authorial comprehension

We could also transfer the authorial comprehension of this book to the dialogue between you, the reader, and me, the writer. Authorial comprehension in both of us occurs when we are guided by questions of how a fact is constituted and what and who "constitutes a fact for me and others; why it is important, for whom, and for what; who cares and why; why I am focusing now on inferring facts and not on something else; and so on" (Matusov, 2015, p. 412).

Authorial comprehension requires that you, the reader, understand what I write with the intention to create a holistic perspective in you. This involves creativity in transcending anything already given to another sphere, one that is both familiar and possibly transformed from the substance of your everyday experience (Matusov, 2015).

For me, the writer, authorial comprehension requires science-in-action, opening up for whatever new meanings could be derived from it. In this way, authorial comprehension becomes a process between us that locates meaning in a dialogical relationship between ones who raise genuine, serious, interested questions. Each person does not know the answer to each question he/she asks, and the other person takes each question seriously and replies to it to the best of his or her knowledge (Matusov, 2015).

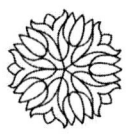

Chapter 16

A RETURN TO THE QUESTION: WHAT IS MUSIC THERAPY?

FRAMING THE QUESTION

In chapter 1, I discussed the troubles connected to the question *What is music therapy?* For my theory on musical answerability to be valuable for foundational thinking in music therapy, I will return to the challenges connected to this basic question.

First, I wish to turn to music therapist and theorist Brynjulf Stige. He thinks that the struggles of creating answers to the basic question can be seen in two ways (Stige, 2003): (1) that it is a practical problem of communication, and (2) that it reveals how the field of music therapy is an emerging field, in continuous change. He therefore supposes that a helpful rephrasing of the question is: What *could* music therapy be?

Stige has a point. Yet I do not believe that a rephrasing of the question solves the dilemmas of the need to try to communicate an essence of the basic question above. Besides, rhetorically, a rephrasing does not make the first question go away. Questions that go beyond this could be: Why does the confidence that music therapists experience in their clinical work crumble away the moment they need to articulate it? Wittgenstein's (1967, p. 42) description of "something that we know when no one asks us but no longer know when we are supposed to give an account of it" is fitting here. Could the amount of tacit and embodied knowledge make it difficult for music therapists to negotiate with other professions what music therapy is?

I wish to approach the question differently. From a rhetorical perspective, does not asking what music therapy is predict that music therapy is *something?* I assume that it is a "something," which, despite the fact that we might have different experiences with music therapy, needs to appear in related ways in music therapists' minds. The hard task, then, is to describe the constants embedded in the experiences and the perceptions connected to the word "what" in the question. Interestingly, the first image that came to mind as I started defining the core concepts in the book was the picture of the video-recorded music therapy improvisation, which is described in the narrative.

Immediately, as the question "What is music therapy?" reached my tongue, the "film" started to run in my mind; I re-experienced, so to speak, the feelings of the music, the actions, the facial gestures, and so on. This experience made me realize that the least important word in the question was "what," while the most important one appeared to be "is." This impulse taught me that the verb and the action word "is" brings forward the vital images of the authentic micro-level, where the music therapy improvisation actually appears and is present and where, for example, the sound of the client is audible and his body/facial expressions visible. I assume that this is the image that I want to communicate to the world outside.

One consequence is that "re-" words, such as re-search, re-present, re-cognition, re-flection, and so forth, which appear *after* the events of the "is," create a contradiction to this realization. The practice of music therapy improvisation remains, in this sense, as Ansdell says, "recalcitrant to discourse" (Ansdell, 1999, p. 420).

Since only action can determine its presence, I am again reminded of the close connection between music therapy improvisation and the phenomenon of action. For me, this also explains why a definition fixed with words on a piece of paper cannot justify the experience of the vital live situation. Going from a present "is" to the sometimes disturbing "what," and from the immediate experience to the verbal and/or oral description, therefore implies, above all, translation of time and perspective. Because theory merely deals with the deterministic components of action, there is a danger of excluding crucial nondeterministic components. This is unfortunate. Therefore, together with Aigen (1991), I question whether a scientific theory built on an unbalanced foundation can address the questions that are relevant to music therapists, who deal with the entire range of human actions.

The traditional scientific view of things is that we treat what we are studying as an object of thought in order to form theories to guide our further deliberate actions in relation to it (Shotter, 1999). Our theories on music therapy and on improvisation are only representations of them that suggest to us ways in which they can be manipulated and give us power over them. "Lacking such pictures, we feel uncertainty, a lack of confidence in our knowledge; we do not quite know where we stand" (Shotter, 1999, p. 18). But the urge for certainty cannot be satisfied in Bakhtin's dialogical universe, for dialogue and the multivoiced polyphony of a world in discussion with itself cannot be framed or theorized (Shotter, 1999, p. 18). Instead of certainty, we might concern ourselves with adequacy, with doing justice to the being of what we are studying (Shotter, 1992). But we cannot expect this transition to be an easy one.

RESPONSIVENESS AND MUSICALLY ANSWERABLE ACTS

I have kept dialogue as an ideal, which sometimes allows monological aspects. Monologism, at its extreme, denies the existence outside itself of another consciousness with equal rights and equal responsibilities, another I with equal rights (You). This is, of course, not what I want. I am sure that it is not what other music therapists want either. "Monologue is finalized and deaf to the other's response, does not expect it, and does not acknowledge it in any decisive force" (Bakhtin, 1984, pp. 292–293).

Our task as music therapists, then, is to construct the Other as a dialogical Being, in a way that we do not objectify him or finalize him. This is a risky operation, but perhaps it must be risky; perhaps we even need to risk being changed ourselves if we want change to happen?

From a Bakhtinian perspective, surrendering to the moment and to our willingness to "other" ourselves is basic in existence. If we allow the otherness to rejoice in us, change might happen as a "bestowed gift" (Bakhtin, 1990, p. 136).

In this book, I have tried to show that risks are worth taking. To become musically answerable acts, our responses are charged by an ethic tension. That is the difficult part, but at the same time, it is the most meaningful part.

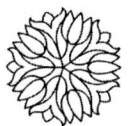

Postlude

The phenomenon of action is in many ways to music therapy improvisation like honey to the bee: Their connection is inevitable, fundamental, and complex, perhaps even too obvious to recognize. Musical answerability has herein been suggested as a theory that embraces this multilayered relationship, and, as we have seen, I have turned to practical as well as philosophical levels of reflection to approach my understanding.

First, I have tried to describe how actions could "behave" within a music therapy improvisation in order to explain its fundamental aspects. As it reveals the bodily based, fragmentary, and prelogical, I have found Bakhtin's metaphor *carnival* to be a suitable illustration for the process. I think that as a practical solution to carnival's idea—which is to actively bring existence down to earth, to where the bodies appear in an unbroken unit—the significance of music therapy improvisation is brought forth.

Music therapy improvisation, as carnival, does not negate the serious. Rather, it purifies and replenishes it, as in serious laughter. Carnival's image therefore fulfils the aim of showing the relevance of both less rational and paradoxical actions in music therapy improvisation. Thus, to frame music therapy improvisation as a phenomenon that includes a range of human actions, this book is an argument for how uncertain aspects could predict a rational outcome in therapy.

Second, for meaning to emerge and develop, which the phenomenon of music therapy improvisation advocates, exploration in a playful condition is crucial. This is above all required to maintain the needed tension between action and intention, which, despite its surprisingly simple illustration, turns out to be the most profound explanation of how the "is" is activated in the question *What is music therapy?*

Also crucial is the dialogical mind-set in the players. This is both typical and necessary for sustaining interest and for the therapy to receive direction. Music creates an exceptional position herein; the inspiration and contentment, which follow from being musically active, help the therapist and the client to direct their actions toward each other.

Seen from an indigenous standpoint, one could say that music therapy improvisation creates a certain type of active togetherness and mastering of dialogical skills, both of which pave the way for therapy. Musical answerability is thus a philosophy about responsiveness in music therapy improvisation and how it becomes a container for change.

The latter seems to be a principle that applies to any music therapy improvisation. Basically, I think that this is independent from developmental level or musical skills. The same mechanisms are found in music therapy improvisations with many clients. One could say that my theory on musical answerability, because it reveals an intuitive form of interplay other than that which is influenced by the early interaction analogy, for example, could reveal how normal interaction could be promoted when the starting point for one of the parties in the relationship is abnormal. In this sense, I think that musical answerability could explain why music is often therapeutically effective.

Because I have chosen an explorative and subjective procedure in my reflection, I have become aware of the crucial limitations that this creates: My text can be a product only of my context center, and I can present it only through the rhetorical nature of my own writing. Nevertheless, I feel that my thinking unifies in particular with music therapy as aesthetic creative theory and social theory, since these are both confronted by the same problem: Both wish for the individual experience to speak.

Words are thus crucial. Yet, words are also fragile (and, as we know, Bakhtin's were almost lost). Translation of language and time is, however, part of the construction job, for both the therapist and the researcher. Interestingly, then, one of the most important personal realizations seems to connect to the word "understanding," which from both Gadamer's and Bakhtin's points of departure requires action and people. In Gadamer's (2003) theory on alethic hermeneutics, it is asserted that understanding involves *coming to an understanding with someone*; in other words, the Other is required. As for Bakhtin, he relates understanding directly to his thinking about dialogue and the existential role of the response therein:

> To some extent, primacy belongs to the response, as the activating principle: It creates the ground for understanding. Understanding comes to fruition only in the response. Understanding and response are dialectically merged and mutually condition each other; one is impossible without the other. (Bakhtin, 1981, p. 282)

In music therapy improvisation, the responsiveness is musically performed. Here, answerability is possible because of the music.

For a therapist, answerability belongs to her responsibility. The client is responsible, too. However, for him, the music therapy improvisation is vital, and for Jakob, it represents a chance for him to collectively shape his identity. Karla too shapes her identity by creating alterity through responding to the unknown. Because this is the only way in which we could all come to an understanding with each other, this also reminds us of the need to continue to act, play, laugh, and discuss. This is also the only way in which we can avoid a final answer, which would be a contradiction to musical answerability as an idea.

NO LAST WORDS

So, finally, do I say what I intend to say in this book? I cannot say for sure. Is the book itself answerable? Indeed, this is not up to me to decide; instead, now the responsibility lies with you, its reader. Remember, however, that there are no last words ...

REFERENCES

Abrams, B. (2011). A relationship-based theory of music therapy: Understanding processes and goals as being-together-musically. In K. Bruscia (Ed.), *Readings in music therapy theory* (pp. 44–64). Gilsum, NH: Barcelona Publishers.

Aigen, K. (1991). *The roots of music therapy: Toward an indigenous research paradigm.* New York, NY: New York University. Ann Arbor, MI: UMI.

Aigen, K. (2005). *Music-Centered Music Therapy.* Gilsum, NH: Barcelona Publishers.

Aksnes, H., & Ruud, E. (2008). Body-based schemata in receptive music therapy. *Musicae Scientiae, 12*(1), 49–74.

Aldridge, D. (1989). Music, Communication, and Medicine: discussion paper. *Journal of the Royal Society of Medicine, 82*(12), 743–746.

Aldridge, D. (2000). *Spirituality, Healing, and Medicine—Return to Silence.* London, UK: Jessica Kingsley.

Aldridge, D. (2001). *Music therapy and neurological rehabilitation: Recognition and the performed body in an ecological niche.* Music Therapy Today: www.musictherapyworld.info.

Alvesson, M., & Sköldberg, K. (2000). *Reflexive Methodology. New Vistas for Qualitative Research.* London, UK: SAGE Publications.

Ansdell, G. (1999). *Music Therapy as Discourse & Discipline, A Study of "Music Therapist's Dilemma."* London, UK: City University, Dept. of Music.

Ansdell, G. (2014). *How Music Helps: A Perspective from Music Therapy.* Aldershot, UK: Ashgate.

Ansdell, G., & Pavlicevic, M. (2005). Musical companionship, musical community. Music therapy and the process and value of musical communication. In D. Miell (Ed.), *Musical Communication* (pp. 193–213). Oxford, UK: Oxford Press.

Bakhtin, M. (1981). *The Dialogic Imagination.* Austin, TX: University of Texas Press.

Bakhtin, M. (1984). *Problems of Dostoevsky's poetics.* Minneapolis, MN: University of Minnesota Press.

Bakhtin, M. (1986a). *Rabelais och skrattets historia.* Uddevalla, Sweden: Bokforlaget Anthropos.

Bakhtin, M. (1986b). *Speech genres and other late essays.* Austin, TX: University of Texas Press.

Bakhtin, M. (1990). *Art and Answerability. Early Philosophical Essays by M. M. Bakhtin.* Austin, TX: University of Texas Press.

Bakhtin, M. M. (1993). *Toward a Philosophy of the Act* (V. Liapunov, Trans.; V. Liapunov & M. Holquist, Eds.). Austin, TX: University of Texas Press.

Bakhtin, M. (2003). *Latter og dialog. Utvalgte skrifter.* Oslo, Norway: Cappelen Akademisk Forlag.

Bateson, G. (1972). *Steps to an Ecology of Mind: Collected Essays in Anthropology, Psychiatry, Evolution, and Epistemology.* Chicago, IL: University of Chicago.

Baxter, L. (2011). *Voicing Relationships. A Dialogic Perspective.* Los Angeles, CA: SAGE.

Blaikie, N. (2003). *Analyzing quantitative data: From description to explanation.* London, UK: SAGE.

Bonde, L. O., Ruud, E., Skånland, M., & Trondalen, G. (2013). *Musical Life Stories. Narratives on Health Musicking.* Series from the Centre for Music and Health, vol. 6 (authors' personal narratives), pp. 263–288. Oslo, Norway: NMH Publications, 2013:5.

Brandist, C. (2011). Foreword. In E. White & A. Peters (Eds.), *Bakhtinian Pedagogy: Opportunities and challenges for research, policy, and practice in education across the globe.* New York, NY: Peter Lang Publishing, Inc.

Bruscia, K. (1987). *Improvisational Models of Music Therapy.* Springfield, IL: Charles C Thomas.

Bruscia, K. (1989). *Defining music therapy.* Gilsum, NH: Barcelona Publishers.

Bruscia, K. (1996). Authenticity Issues in Qualitative Research. In M. Langenberg, K. Aigen, & J. Frommer (Eds.), *Qualitative Music Therapy Research. Beginning Dialogue* (pp. 81–107). Gilsum, NH: Barcelona Publishers.

Bruscia, K. (1998). *Defining music therapy* (2nd ed.). Gilsum, NH: Barcelona Publishers.

Bruscia, K. (2000). The Nature of Meaning in Music Therapy. (Bruscia interviewed by Brynjulf Stige). *Nordic Journal of Music Therapy, 9*(2).

Bruscia, K. (2005). Developing Theory. In B. Wheeler (Ed.), *Music Therapy Research* (pp. 540–551). Gilsum, NH: Barcelona Publishers.

Bruscia, K. (2014). *Defining music therapy* (3rd ed.). Gilsum, NH: Barcelona Publishers.

Buber, M. (1992). *Jeg og du.* Oslo, Norway: Cappelens forlag.

Børtnes, J. (2001). Bakhtin, dialogen, og den andre. In O. Dysthe (Ed.), *Dialog, samspel, og læring.* Oslo, Norway: Abstrakt Forlag.

Christophersen, C. (2009). *Rytmisk musikkundervisning som estetisk praksis: en casestudie* (PhD thesis). Norwegian Academy of Music. Oslo, Norway: NMH Publications, 2009:2.

Clark, K., & Holquist, M. (1984). *Mikhail Bakhtin.* Cambridge, MA: Belknap Press of Harvard Univ. Press.

Csikszentmihalyi, M. (1990). *Flow. The Psychology of Optimal Experience.* New York, NY: Harper Perennial.

Dryden, D. (2004). *Susanne K. Langer.* Durham, NC: Duke University. Retrieved Oct. 20, 2015, from http://www.huthsteiner.org/Knauth/Susanne.Knath.Langer_Bio_DLB.pdf

Emerson, C. (2000). *The first hundred years of Mikhail Bakhtin.* Princeton, NJ: Princeton Univ. Press.

Ferrara, L. (1984). Phenomenology as a tool for Musical Analyses. *The Musical Quarterly, 70*(3), 355–373.

Frønes, I. (1995). *Handling og sosial struktur (1 og 2).* Oslo, Norway: Univ. of Oslo, Dep. of Sociology.

Gadamer, H.-G. (2003). *Truth and Method.* New York, NY: The Continuum Publishing Company.

Garred, R. (2004). *Dialogical Dimensions of Music Therapy. Framing the Possibility of a Music-based Therapy* (PhD thesis). Inst. of Music and Music Therapy. Aalborg, Denmark: Aalborg Univ.

Garred, R. (2006). *Music as Therapy: A Dialogical Perspective.* Gilsum, NH: Barcelona Publishers.

Hauge, T. S., & Tønsberg, G. E. H. (1996). The Musical Nature of Prelinguistic Interaction. *Nordic Journal of Music Therapy, 5*(2), 63–75.

Hauge, T. S., & Tønsberg, G. E. H. (1998). *Musikalske aspekter i førspråkelig samspill. En analyse av musikalske elementer mellom døvblindfødte barn og seende hørende voksne.* Oslo, Norway: Skådalen kompetansesenter.

Hellendoorn, J., van der Kooij, R., & Sutton-Smith, B. (Eds.). (1994). *Play and Intervention.* Albany, NY: State University of New York Press.

Hirschkop, K. (1990). *Mikhail Bakhtin: An aesthetic for Democracy.* Oxford, UK: Oxford Univ. Press.

Holck, U. (2002). *"Kommunikalsk" samspill i musikterapi. Kvalitative videoanalyser af musikalske og gestiske interaktioner med børn med betydelige funktionsnedsættelser, herunder børn med autisme* (PhD thesis). Inst. for Musik og Musikterapi. Aalborg, Denmark: Aalborg Univ.

Holck, U. (2004). Interaction Themes in Music Therapy: Definition and Delimitation. *Nordic Journal of Music Therapy, 13*(1), 3–19.

Holquist, M. (1990). *Dialogism, Bakhtin, and his World.* London, UK: Routledge.

Horgen, T. (2010). Musikk, helse, multifunksjonshemming. In K. Stensæth, A. T. Eggen, & R. S. Frisk (Eds.), *Musikk, helse, multifunksjonshemming* (pp. 5–22), Oslo, Norway: Norwegian Academy of Music, Series from the Centre for Music and Health, vol. 3.

Juxwik, M. (2004). *Towards an Ethics of Answerability: Reconsidering Dialogism in Sociocultural Literacy Research.* The National Council of Teachers of English. Retrieved June 1, 2017, from http://juzwik.wiki.educ.msu.edu/file/view/Juzwik_2004_CCC.pdf

Kanellopoulos, P. (2011a). In pursuit of Musical Freedom Through Free Improvisation: A Bakhtinian Provocation to Music Education. In J. E. White & A. Peters (Eds.), *Bakhtinian Pedagogy: Opportunities and Challenges for Research, Policy, and Practice in Education Across the Globe* (pp. 91–116). New York, NY: Peter Lang Publishing, Inc.

Kanellopoulos, P. (2011b). Freedom and responsibility. The aesthetics of free musical improvisation and its educational implications—a view from Bakhtin. *Philosophy of Music Education Reviews, 19*(2), 113–135.

Keil, C. (1995). The theory of participatory discrepancies: A progress report. *Ethnomusicology, 39*(1), 1–20.

Keil, C., & Feld, S. (1994). *Music grooves: essays and dialogues.* Chicago, IL: University of Chicago Press.

Kenny, C. B. (1987/1988). *The field of play: A theoretical study of music therapy process.* Santa Barbara, CA: The Fielding Institute.

Kenny, C. B. (1989). *The field of play: a guide for the theory and practice of music therapy.* Atascadero, CA: Ridgeview Pub. Co.

Kenny, C. B. (1995). *Listening, playing, creating: essays on the power of sound.* Albany, NY: State University of New York Press.

Kenny, C. B. (2005). Narrative Inquiry. In B. Wheeler (Ed.), *Music Therapy Research* (pp. 416–428). Gilsum, NH: Barcelona Publishers.

Keunen, B. (2011). *Time and Imagination: Chronotopes in Western Narrative Culture.* Evanston, IL: Northwestern University Press.

Kruse, B. (2016). *Thinking Art. An Interdisciplinary Approach to Applied Aesthetics.* NMH Publications, 2016:2, NordArt (Arne Nordheim Centre for Artistic Research), vol. 1. Oslo, Norway: Norwegian Academy of Music.

Kvernbekk, T. (2005). *Pedagogisk teoridannelse. Insidere, teoriformer og praksis.* Bergen, Norway: Fagbokforlaget.

Langer, S. K. (1952). *Philosophy in a New Key.* New York, NY: Mentor.

Langer, S. K. (1953/1977). *Feeling and Form.* New York, NY: Charles Scribner's Sons.

Leiman, M. (2011). Mikhail Bakhtin's contribution to psychotherapy research. *Culture & Psychology, 17*(4), 441–461. doi:10.1177/1354067X11418543

Leontjev, A. N. (1977). *Problemer med det psykiskes udvikling* (Bind 3). Copenhagen, Denmark: Rhodos.

Levinas, E. (1989). Ethics as first philosophy. In S. Hand (Ed.), *The Levinas reader* (pp. 75–87). Oxford, UK: Blackwell.

Levinas, E. (1998). *On thinking-of-the-other.* London, UK: Athlone.

Lillis, T. (2003). Student writing as "academic literacies": Drawing on Bakhtin to move from critique to design. *Language and Education, 17*(3), 192–207.

Lorentzen, P. (2001). *Uvanlige barns språk.* Oslo, Norway: Universitetsforlaget.

Malloch, S., & Trevarthen, C. (Eds.). (2009). *Communicative Musicality. Exploring the Basis of Human Companionship.* Oxford, UK: Oxford University Press.

Marková, I. (2003). Constitution of the self: Intersubjectivity and dialogicality. *Culture & Psychology, 9*(3), 249-259.

Martinsen, K. (2003). *Fra Marx til Løgstrup: om etikk og sanselighet i sykepleien.* Oslo, Norway: Universitetsforlaget.

Martinsen, K. (2005). *Samtalen, skjønnet og evidensen.* Oslo, Norway: Akribe.

Matusov, E. (2001). Intersubjectivity as a way of informing teaching design for a community of learners classroom. *Teaching and Teacher Education, 17,* 383-402. Newark, DE: Univ. of Delaware, School of Education.

Matusov, E. (2009). *Journey into Dialogic Pedagogy.* New York, NY: Nova Science Publishers, Inc.

Matusov, E. (2010). Bakhtin's notion of the internally persuasive discourse in education. In K. Junefely & P. Nordin (Eds.), *Proceedings from the Second International Interdisciplinary Conference on Perspectives and Limits of Dialogism in Mikhail Bakhtin* (pp. 174-199). Stockholm, Sweden: Stockholm Univ.

Matusov, E. (2011). Authorial teaching and learning. In E. J. White & M. Peters (Eds.), *Bakhtinian Pedagogy: Opportunities and challenges for research, policy, and practice in education across the globe* (pp. 21-46). New York, NY: Peter Lang Publishers.

Matusov, E. (2015). Comprehension: A dialogic authorial approach. *Culture & Psychology, 21*(3), 392-416. doi:10.1177/1354067X15601197

Mead, G. H. (1962). *Mind, Self, and Society.* Chicago, IL: University of Chicago Press.

Morson, G. S., & Emerson, C. (1990). *Mikhail Bakhtin. Creation of a Prosaics.* Stanford, CA: Stanford Univ. Press.

Murray, J. (2009). Bakhtinian answerability and Levinasian responsibility: Forging a fuller dialogical communicative ethics. *Southern Communication Journal, 65*(2-3), 133-150. doi:10.1080/1+417940009373163

Nordenfelt, L. (1991). *Hälsa och värde.* Stockholm, Sweden: Bokförlaget Thales.

Nordoff, P., & Robbins, C. (1965). *Music therapy for handicapped children; investigations and experiences.* New York, NY: R. Steiner Publications.

Nordoff, P., & Robbins, C. (1971a). *Music therapy in special education.* New York, NY: John Day Co.

Nordoff, P., & Robbins, C. (1971b). *Therapy in music for handicapped children.* New York, NY: St. Martin's Press.

Nordoff, P., & Robbins, C. (1977). *Creative Music Therapy. Individual Treatment for the Handicapped Child.* New York, NY: John Day Co.

Nordoff, P., & Robbins, C. (1985). *Therapy in music for handicapped children.* London, UK: Gollancz.

Pampa, O. A. (2014). The question of the author in Bakhtin. *Bakhtiniana, Rev. Estud. Discurso*, vol. 9. Retrieved March 27, 2017, from http://www.scielo.br/ scielo.php?pid=S2176-45732014000300002&script= sci_arttext&tlng=en

Pavlicevic, M. (1997). *Music therapy in context: Music, meaning, and relationship* London, UK, & Philadelphia, PA: Jessica Kingsley Publishers.

Pavlicevic, M. (2000). Improvisation in Music Therapy: Human Communication in Sound. *Journal of Music Therapy, 37*(4), 269–285.

Pavlicevic, M. (2002). Dynamic Interplay in Clinical Improvisation. *Voices: A World Forum for Music Therapy:* www.voices.no/mainissues.

Pavlicevic, M., & Ansdell, G. (2009). "Between communicative musicality and collaborative musicking: A perspective from communicative music therapy." In S. Malloch & C. Trevarthen (Eds.), *Communicative Musicality. Exploring the Basis of Human Companionship* (pp. 357–376). Oxford, UK: Oxford University Press.

Poole, B. (1998). "Bakhtin and Cassirer": The Philosophical Origins of Bakhtin's Carnival Messianism. *South Atlantic Quarterly, 97*(3–4), 542–544.

Ruud, E. (1980). *Music Therapy and its Relationship to Current Treatment Theories.* St. Louis, MO: Magnamusic Baton.

Ruud, E. (1996). *Musikk og verdier.* Oslo, Norway: Universitetsforlaget.

Ruud, E. (1998). *Music therapy: improvisation, communication, and culture.* Gilsum, NH: Barcelona Publishers.

Ruud, E. (2010). *Music therapy. A Perspective from the Humanities.* Gilsum, NH: Barcelona Publishers.

Ruud, E. (2016). *Musikkvitenska*p. Oslo, Norway: Universitetsforlaget.

Schatzki, T. R. (2001). Introduction: Practice theory. In T. R Schatzki, K. K. Cetina, & E. v. Savigny (Eds.), *The Practice Turn in Contemporary Theory* (pp. 10–23). London, UK: Routledge.

Schei, E. (2009). Helsebegrepet—selvet og cellen. In E. Ruud (Ed.), *Musikk i psykisk helsearbeid med barn og unge* (pp. 7–15). Series from the Centre for Music and Health, vol. 2. Oslo, Norway: Norwegian Academy of Music.

Schiller, F. (1967). *On the Aesthetic Education of Man in a Series of Letters* (E. M. Wilkinson & L. A. Willoughby, Eds. & Trans.). Oxford, UK: Clarendon Press.

Schön, D. A. (1983). *The reflective practitioner: How professionals think in action.* New York, NY: Basic Books.

Schütz, A. (1951). Making music together. *Social Research, 18,* 76–97.

Shepherd, D. (1998). *The Contexts of Bakhtin: Philosophy, Authorship, Aesthetics.* Routledge Harwood Studies in Russian and European Literature. London, UK: Routledge.

Shotter, J. (1992). Bakhtin and Billig. Monological Versus Dialogical Practices. *American Behavioral Scientist, 36*(1), 8–21. SAGE Publications.

Shotter, J. (1999). Life inside dialogically structured mentalities: Bakhtin's and Voloshinov's account of our mental activities as out in the world between us. In J. Rowan & M. Cooper (Eds.), *The Plural Self* (pp. 71–92). London, UK: SAGE Publications.

Skårberg, O. (1998). Musikkterapi som estetisk praksis: Noen refleksjoner omkring musikk- og handlingsbegreper. *Nordisk tidsskrift for musikkterapi, 7*(1), 24–34.

Skjervheim, H. (1996). *Deltakar og tilskodar og andre essays.* Oslo, Norway: Aschehoug.

Slaatelid, R. T. (1998). *Bakhtins translingvestikk. Spørsmålet om talegenrane.* Bergen, Norway: Ariadne Forlag.

Steinsholt, K. (1998). *Lett som en lek?* Trondheim, Norway: Tapir Forlag.

Stensæth, K. (2002). *"Musikkterapi som kjær-leik." Kva kan leiken seie om musikkterapeutisk improvisasjon? Ei grunnlagsfilosofisk drøfting.* Master's thesis, Institute for Music and Theater. Oslo, Norway: Univ. of Oslo.

Stensæth, K. (2006). *"Det dialogiske menneske." Mikhail Bakhtin sin dialogfilosofi; Eit mogeleg perspektiv for musikkterapeuten?* Flerstemmige Innspill. NMH-publications. Oslo, Norway: Norwegian Academy of Music.

Stensæth, K. (2008). *Musical Answerability. A Theory on the Relationship Between Music Therapy Improvisation and the Phenomenon of Action* (PhD thesis, Norwegian Academy of Music). Oslo, Norway: NMH Publications, 2008:2.

Stensæth, K. (2013). Musical Co-creation? Exploring health-promoting potentials on the use of musical and interactive tangibles for families with children with disabilities. *International Journal of Qualitative Studies on Health and Well-being, MS ID: 20704, Special Issue on Music and Health* (no paging).

Stensæth, K. (2015). "Musical dialoguing": A perspective of Bakhtin's Dialogue on musical improvisation in asymmetric relations. In E. Georgii-Hemming, S.-E. Holgersen, Ø. Varkøy, & L. Väkevä (Eds.), *Nordic Research in Music Education Yearbook*, vol. 16 (pp. 209–226). Oslo, Norway: Norwegian Academy of Music.

Stensæth, K. (2017). "Nye handlemuligheter" gjennom handling? In K. Stensæth, G. Trondalen, & Ø. Varkøy (Eds.), *Musikk og handlemuligheter. Festskrift til Even Ruud* (pp. 55–68), Oslo, Norway: Norwegian Academy of Music, Series from CREMAH, vol. 10.

Stensæth, K., & Eide, I. B. (2016). Umberto Eco's notions of the "open work" and the "field of possibilities": New perspectives on music therapy and co-creation? *British Journal of Music Therapy*, 1–11. doi: 10.1177/1359457516678622

Stensæth, K., & Næss, T. (2013). "Together!" RagnaRock, the Band, and Their Musical Life Story. In L. O. Bonde, E. Ruud, M. Skånland, & G. Trondalen (Eds.), *Musical Life Stories. Narratives on Health Musicking.* Series from the Centre for Music and Health, vol. 6 (pp. 263–288). Oslo, Norway: NMH Publications, 2013:5.

Stensæth, K., & Ruud, E. (2014). An interactive technology for health: New possibilities for the field of music and health and for music therapy? A case study of two children with disabilities playing with "ORFI." In K. Stensæth (Ed.), *Music, Health, Technology, and Design.* Series from the Centre for Music and Health, vol. 8 (pp. 39–66). Oslo, Norway: Norwegian Academy of Music.

Stern, D. (2000). *Barnets interpersonelle verden.* Copenhagen, Denmark: Hans Reitzels Forlag.

Stige, B. (2002). *Culture-centered Music Therapy.* Gilsum, NH: Barcelona Publishers.

Stige, B. (2003). "What Could Music Therapy Be?" *Voices: A World Forum for Music Therapy:* www.voices.no/mainissues.

Stige, B. (2015). The practice turn in music therapy theory. *Music Therapy Perspectives, 33*(1), 1–8.

Trevarthen, C. (1989). Infants trying to talk; how a child invites communication from the human world. In R. Søderberg (Ed.), *Children's Creative Communication.* Lund, Sweden: Lund Univ. Press.

Trondalen, G. (2004). *Klingende relasjoner. En musikkterapistudie av "signifikante øyeblikk" i musikalsk samspill med unge mennesker med anoreksi.* Oslo, Norway: Norwegian Academy of Music.

Trondalen, G. (2016). *Relational music therapy. An Intersubjective Perspective.* Dallas, TX: Barcelona Publishers.

Tufte, T. (2011). *Fra teori til handling. Om skjønn i en evidensbasert praksis.* Master's thesis, Department of Social Studies, Oslo and Akershus University College of Applied Sciences. Retrieved August 20, 2016, from https://oda.hio.no/jspui/bitstream/10642/920/2/Tufte_Turid.pdf

Turner, V. (1969). *The ritual process: structure and antistructure.* Ithaca, NY: Cornell University Press.

Tønsberg, G. E. H. (2010). Improvisasjon i et dialogisk kommunikasjonsperspektiv. In K. Stensæth, A. T. Eggen, & R. S. Frisk (Eds.), *Musikk, helse, multifunksjonshemming.* Series from the Centre for Music and Health, vol. 3 (pp. 41–54). Oslo, Norway: Norwegian Academy of Music.

Tønsberg, G. E. H., & Hauge, T. S. (2003). The musical nature of human interaction. *Voices: A World Forum for Music Therapy:* www.voices.no/mainissues.

Wetherell, M. (2001). Minds, Selves, and Sense Making (Editor's Introduction). In M. Wetherell, S. Taylor, & S. J. Yates, (Eds.), *Discourse Theory and Practice* (pp. 186–197). London, UK: SAGE Publications Ltd.

White, E., & Peters, A. (Eds.). (2011). *Bakhtinian Pedagogy: Opportunities and challenges for research, policy, and practice in education across the globe.* New York, NY: Peter Lang Publishing, Inc.

Wigram, T. (2004). *Improvisation. Methods and Techniques for Music Therapy Clinicians, Educators, and Students.* London, UK: Jessica Kingsley Publishers.

Wittgenstein, L. (1967). *Philosophical investigations.* Oxford, UK: Basil Blackwell.

Østerberg, D. (1993). *Fortolkende sosiologi I.* Oslo, Norway: Universitetsforlaget (Det blå bibiliotek).

Østerberg, D. (1997). *Fortolkende sosiologi II.* Oslo, Norway: Universitetsforlaget (Det blå bibliotek).

Østerberg, D. (2003). *Sosiologiens nøkkelbegreper.* Oslo, Norway: Cappelen Akademisk Forlag.

Østerberg, D., & Bjørnerheim, R. T. (2017). *Musikkfeltet. Innføring i musikksosiologi.* Oslo, Norway: Cappelen Damm Akademisk.

ATTACHMENTS

THE GUITAR EXCERPT

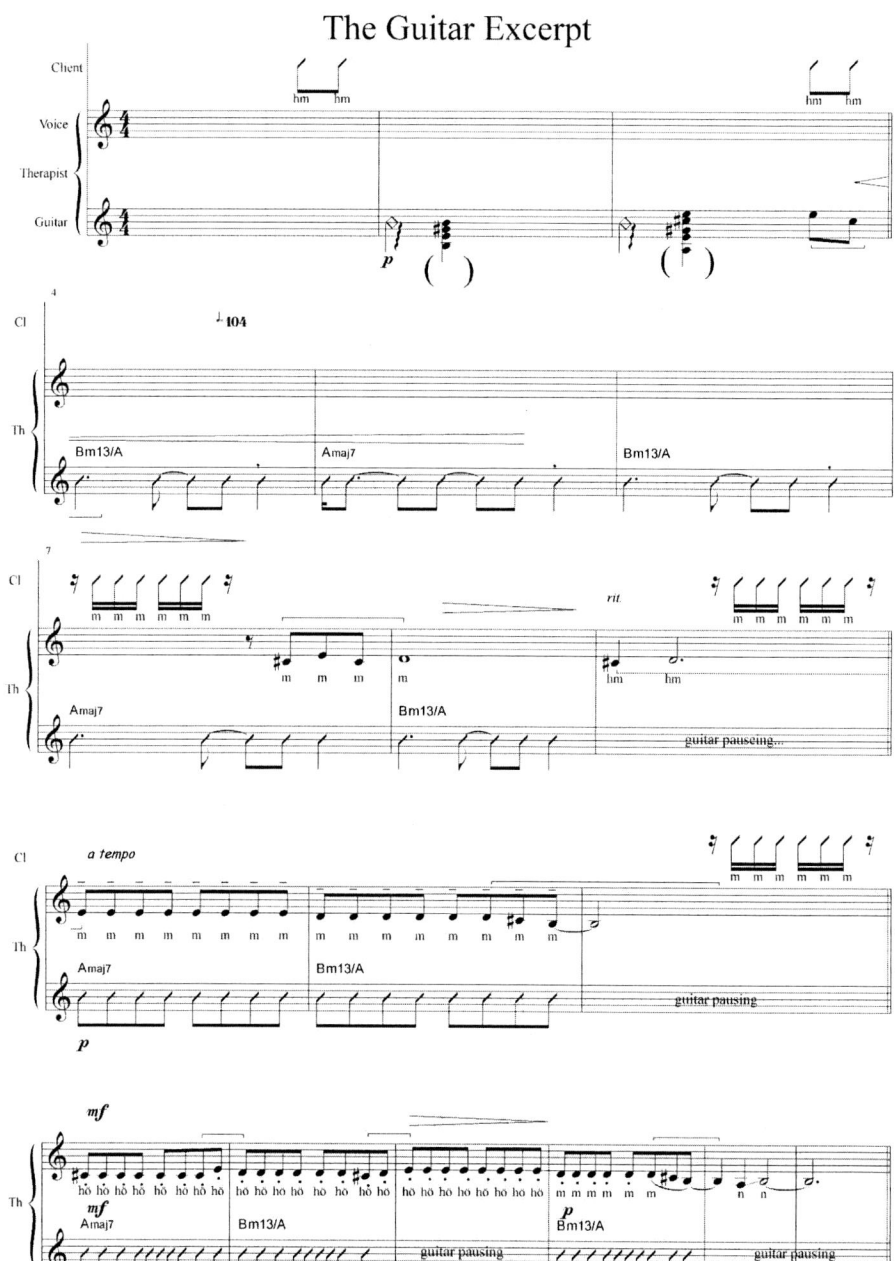

The Guitar Excerpt, part 2

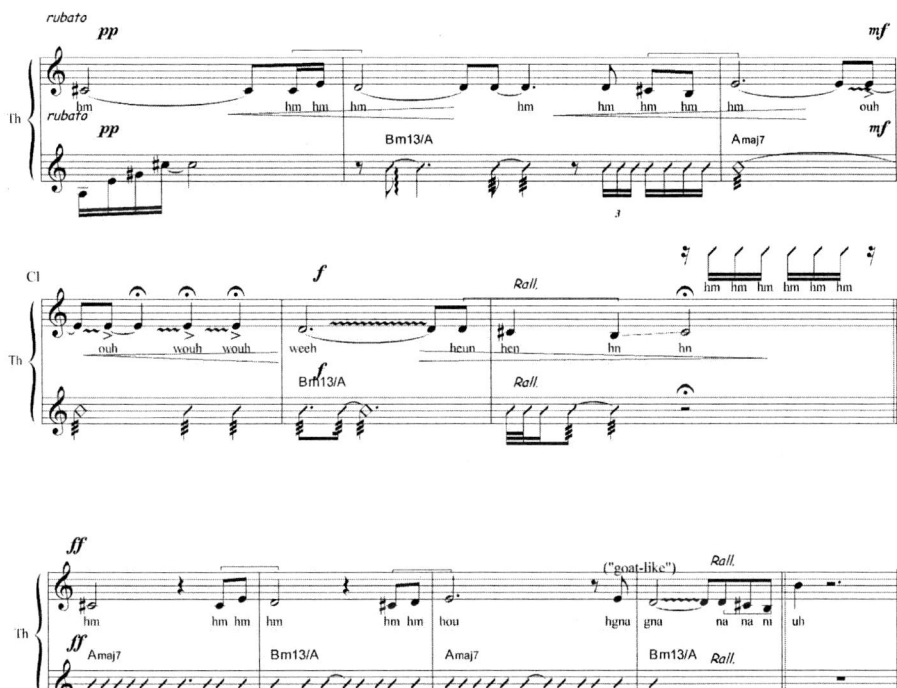

THE DJEMBE EXCERPT

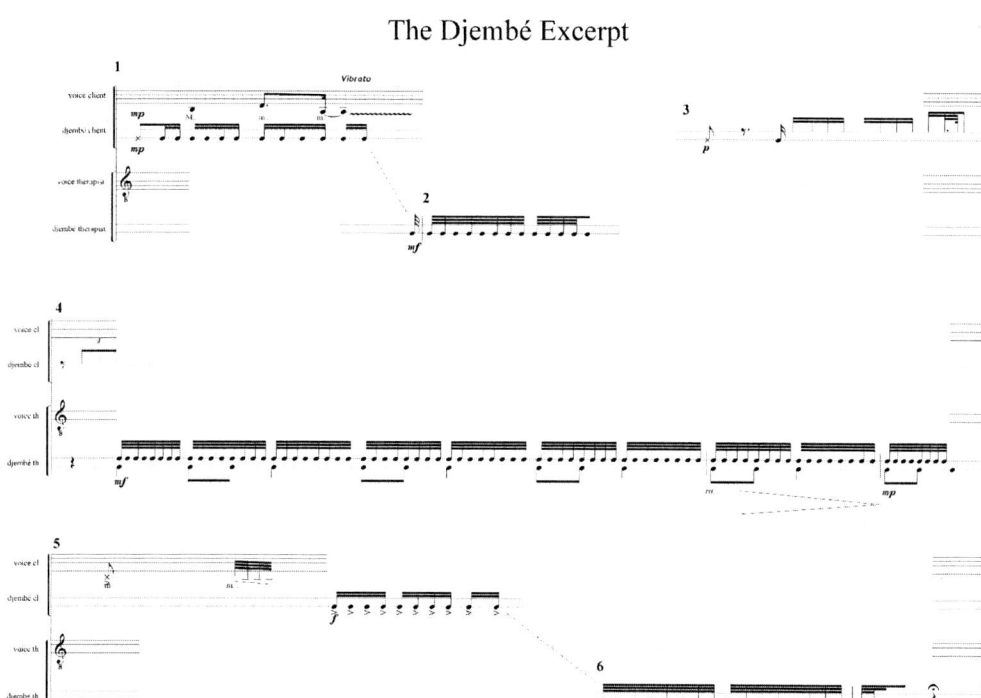

The Djembe Excerpt, part 2

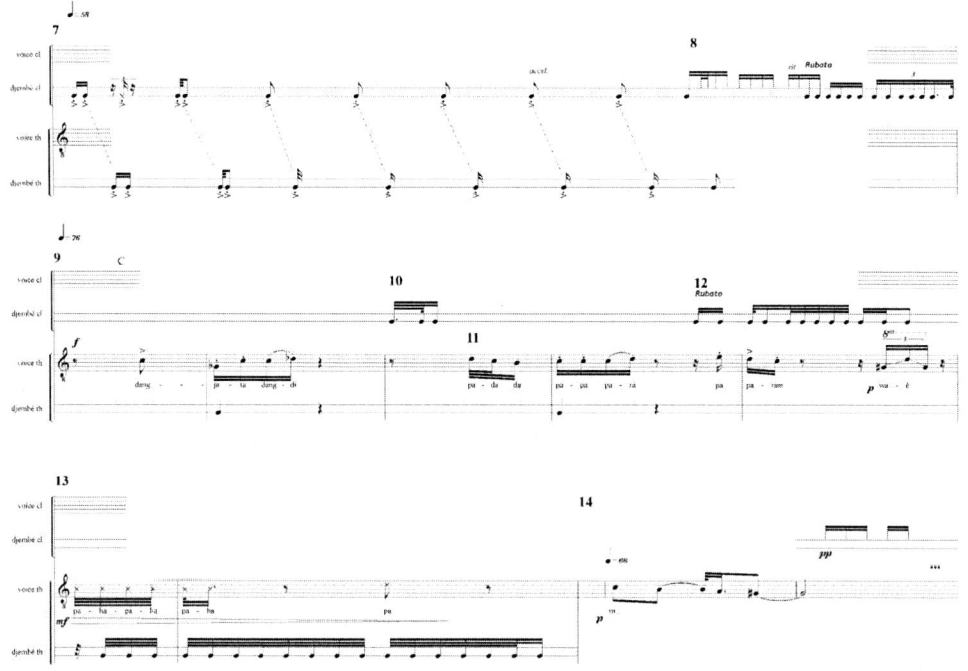

THE DJEMBE EXCERPT, PART 3

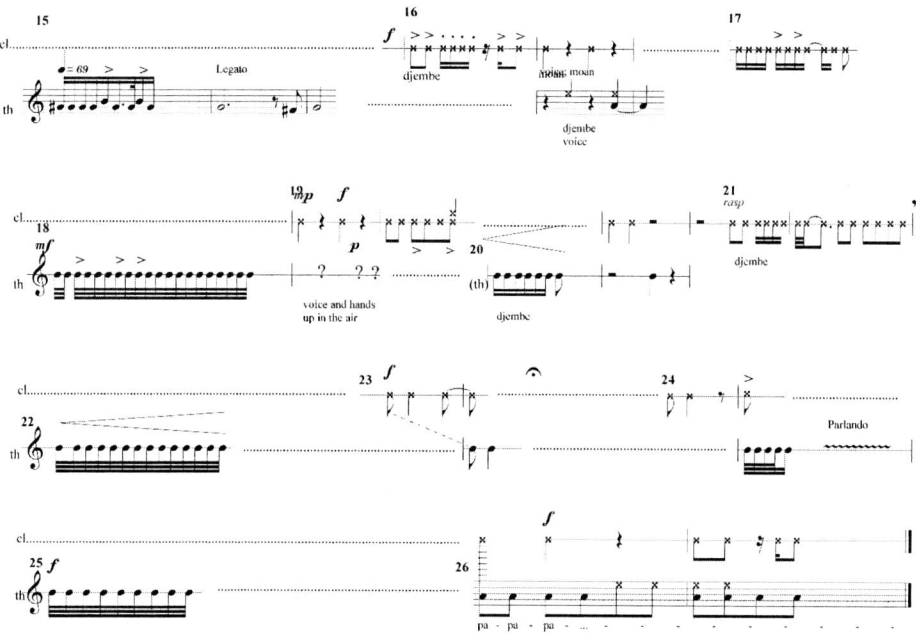

ENDNOTES

1. Brandist is a professor of cultural theory and intellectual history at the University of Sheffield.
2. Matusov is a professor of education in the School of Education at the University of Delaware.
3. Retrieved March 18, 2017, from https://en.wikipedia.org/wiki/Ecole_d'Humanit%C3%A9
4. Retrieved March 18, 2017, from https://en.wikipedia.org/wiki/Ernst_Cassirer
5. Retrieved May 26, 2017, from http://www.thesaurus.com/browse/responsiveness?s=t
6. Bruscia (1987) has written more than 500 pages about the different improvisational models in music therapy.
7. I write "Other" with a capital O when I refer to Bakhtin's use of the term "Other."
8. For simplicity, and to correspond with the genders of the client and the therapist in the narrative, the music therapist will be referred to as female and the client as male.
9. It is in her understanding of art as symbolism that Langer is inspired by Cassirer, the philosopher who in turn inspired Paul and Edith Geheeb, the founders of "my" school, École d'Humanité. See the Introduction.
10. I have translated the citations of Frønes and Østerberg. Also, my presentation of Østerberg's theories refers in a major way to another article I wrote (Stensæth, 2017).
11. The setting when the music therapy took place also involved Jakob's caretaker. She knew Jakob better than I did. She would assist him by holding an instrument for him and by comforting him when needed.
12. Retrieved Jan. 6, 2017, from https://en.wikipedia.org/wiki/Heteroglossia
13. Read more about this at https://deontologistics.files.wordpress.com/2012/01/levinas.pdf
14. Trondalen (2016) uses Levinas to describe her perspective on intersubjectivity.
15. Kanellopoulos refers to several other writings of Bakhtin here.
16. Retrieved April 1, 2017, from https://hhs.hud.ac.uk
17. Much of this paragraph is collected from other articles I have written (Stensæth, 2006, 2015).
18. This part brings back memories from my time in the École d'Humanité in 1978-79, and the school's motto "Become Who You Are." Probably, I experienced something like a We-community built on the musical togetherness in the school's choir rehearsal (read my personal narrative in the Introduction).
19. The term "close other" is used by several people in disability research (e.g., Horgen, 2010; Stensæth & Eide, 2016).

20. Janus was an ancient Roman god of doorways, of beginnings, and of the rising and setting of the Sun and was usually represented as having one head with two bearded faces back to back, looking in opposite directions, one young and one old. Consequently, a hypocritical person is often called "Janus-faced" (retrieved Sept. 7, 2011, from http://dictionary.reference.com/browse/Janus).
21. This point could resemble Csikszentmihalyi's (1990) theories on flow.
22. The citation is verbalized by one of the music therapists observing the video recording.
23. See the whole excerpt in the scores in the attachments.
24. Retrieved August 31, 2007, from http://dictionary.reference.com/browse/exist
25. Retrieved Sept. 7, 2007, from http://dictionary.reference.com/browse/communication
26. Interestingly, this could remind us of the old Greek concept of "muse," which describes how we express ourselves aesthetically and creatively through both bodies and minds as a whole.

INDEX

A

act, 17, 30, 45, 48, 50, 83, 108, 110–12, 114, 135–37, 143, 145, 152, 155–59, 173
action and intention, 40, 44–46, 67, 69–70, 110, 136, 141, 147, 158, 160, 163, 168, 171
actions, types of, 29, 35–36, 43, 132, 134, 155
aesthetics, 13, 24, 29, 33–36, 81, 91, 98, 123–24, 152, 178, 180
air, 59, 63–64, 74, 100, 110, 134, 140, 143, 155
answerability, 37, 81–83, 85, 95, 98, 107–9, 111–13, 115, 117, 156–57, 160, 173, 175, 177
attention, 35, 38, 42, 50–51, 53, 57, 68, 84–86, 133, 137, 140, 142, 145–46, 159, 162

B

Bakhtinian Pedagogy, 74, 176, 178–79, 183
Bakhtin scholars, xiv, 73–77, 82, 90
Bakhtin's Ideas on Answerability, 109, 111, 113, 115
Bakhtin's Ideas on Carnival, 8, 95, 128–33, 137, 139–41, 143, 145–47, 151
Bakhtin's ideas on dialogue, 75, 79, 107, 113, 120, 169
Bakhtin's Ideas on Dialogue Transposed to Responsiveness, 78, 85, 87, 97, 99, 101, 103, 105, 156, 181
Bakhtin's philosophy, 4, 13, 45, 77, 81, 89, 99, 105–7, 112, 169
Bakhtin's Terminology, 81, 83, 85, 87, 89, 91, 93, 95
Bakhtin's world, 125, 127, 137, 150, 153
beat, 31–32, 55, 61–64, 68, 138–39
beauty, 26–27, 29, 35–36
body, 28, 30, 55, 59, 65, 67, 78, 92–93, 97, 110, 153, 155, 164, 168, 171
body language, 67, 78–79
boundaries, 19, 86–87, 105, 146

C

children, 6–8, 25, 47, 122, 129–30, 181–82
chronos, 30, 137
chronos and kairos, 30, 137
chronotope, 90, 147, 160, 178
communication, 18–19, 23, 27–28, 39–40, 66, 68–69, 78–79, 83, 101–2, 104–5, 151, 153–54, 156, 180, 182
community, 10, 31–33, 42, 75, 117–18, 153, 155, 158, 175, 179
consciousnesses, 25–26, 33, 35, 82, 89, 91, 99–100, 103, 109, 114, 118, 123, 136–37, 146, 152
contentment, 47–48, 135–36, 172
Creative Music Therapy, 19, 156, 179
creativity, 18, 83, 91, 93, 128, 158, 161, 165
culture, 5, 9–10, 29, 31, 36, 53, 94, 104, 115, 151, 157, 179–80

D

Defining Core Concepts, 13, 15, 17, 19, 21, 23, 25, 27, 29, 31, 33, 35, 37
defining music therapy, 14–15, 41, 176
development, 13, 15, 21, 26–27, 40–41, 62, 73, 89, 109, 122, 129
dialogical, 86, 99, 101–2, 107, 115, 119–20, 123–24, 142, 150, 155, 161, 175–76
dialogical mind-set, 99, 119–20, 141–43, 159, 172
dialogical processes, 29, 87, 91, 98–99, 105, 114–15, 119, 131, 141, 145, 150–51, 161, 164–65, 177, 179
dialogical theory, 99, 101, 103, 105, 115, 118, 120, 122, 150–51
dialogue
real-life, 87, 97–98

types of, 15, 29, 68, 119, 142
discourses, 88–89, 111, 119, 160, 165
djembe, 60–65, 68, 97–98, 100, 139
Djembe Excerpt, 49, 54, 60–63, 68, 138, 186–88

E

ethics, xiii, 13, 36–37, 81, 98, 104, 121, 124, 151, 155, 178
event, 10–11, 13, 30, 35, 50, 53, 81, 94, 114–15, 138–41, 144–46, 152–53, 163, 168
existence, 78, 84–85, 94, 99–100, 112–13, 153, 156, 169, 171

F

freedom
  expressive, 18, 20–21, 128
  musical, 109, 111–12, 178

G

gestures, 29, 57, 67, 78–79, 97, 105, 110
Guitar Excerpt, 49, 54–56, 59–60, 68, 101, 132–33, 137, 140, 142, 144–45, 184–85

H

health, 11, 14–17, 117, 146, 176–77, 180–82
here-and-now, xiii, 25, 30, 37, 44–45, 98–99, 115, 130, 150, 152, 156, 158
heteroglossia, 88, 111, 164, 189

I

image, 16, 19, 26, 47, 51–52, 57, 79, 86, 97–98, 101, 143, 149, 152–53, 156, 168
immersion, 37, 111–12, 114
impulses, 19, 111, 132, 164–65, 168
infants, 40–41, 121, 133–34, 138, 182
initiative, 16, 41, 57, 60–61, 64–67, 70, 141, 145

inspiration and contentment, 47–48, 135, 172
intention, 28–29, 36, 38, 42, 44–48, 67, 70, 122, 136, 140–41, 147, 155–56, 158, 163, 165
  expressive, 46, 86, 110, 118
interaction, 28–31, 33, 36–37, 50, 60, 62–63, 66, 68–71, 98, 122, 130–31, 133, 138–41, 143, 145
  musical, 25, 41, 51, 60–62, 109, 137
interresponsiveness, 20–21, 157
intersubjectivity, 105, 156, 179, 189

J

joy, 6, 8, 11, 22, 47, 66, 69, 92, 95, 127, 129, 160
judgment, personal, 37, 163

K

kairos, 30, 137
knowledge, 3, 5, 9, 37, 91, 122, 151, 161, 165, 169

L

language, 23, 51, 75, 77–79, 85–88, 94, 146, 172, 178
laughter, 8, 11, 22, 81, 92–93, 95, 127, 171
levels of consciousness, 136–37
life, xiii–xiv, 6, 8–11, 15, 75, 78, 81, 90–94, 99–100, 122, 124, 127, 134, 149–52, 159
logs, 49, 51–54, 97, 101, 133, 139, 143, 163

M

meaning, 13–14, 16, 27–30, 40–42, 45–46, 87–88, 90, 94, 101–2, 115–16, 128–29, 147, 149–56, 158–60, 164–65
  musical, 28–29
minds, 40, 43, 45, 48, 51–52, 104, 106–7, 114, 116, 121–22, 133–34, 152, 155, 168, 176

monologue, 99, 114, 119, 169
motivation, 6–8, 22, 24, 48, 158
musical actions, 3, 24, 102, 141, 144, 149, 154, 156
musical answerability, 3, 150–57, 159–63, 167, 171–73, 181
musicality, communicative, 31, 121, 179–80
Musical Life Stories, 10, 176, 182
Musical-Relational Answerability, 111
musical-relational synchronizing, 69, 153, 157
musical skills, developing, 20–21, 157
musical time, 30
musical utterances, 98, 101, 110, 160
music and health, 176–77, 180–82
music child, 19, 157
music therapy, redefine, 14–15, 17
music therapy theorists, 11, 15, 47, 78, 140, 157, 175, 182
mutuality, 31–32, 85–86

N

Narratives, 8, 10, 52–53, 71, 176, 182
Nordoff & Robbins, 7, 18–20, 22–23, 27, 154, 179

O

obligation, 81, 95, 104, 109–11
observations, 49–53, 64, 66, 70, 138–39, 141–42, 144–45
oughtness, 108–9, 114
outsideness, 113–14, 152

P

playfulness, 18, 36, 128, 135, 137, 139, 141, 143, 145, 147
playing, xiii, 31–32, 47, 50, 58, 62–65, 68, 100–102, 107–10, 115, 118–19, 131, 133, 137, 139–40

R

relation, 4, 7, 18–19, 22, 40–41, 64, 66, 75, 77, 85–86, 108–10, 120–21, 123, 125, 162–63
responsibility, 10, 37, 82, 104–5, 107–9, 112–13, 133, 149, 173–74, 178
Responsiveness and Musically Answerable Acts, 19, 23, 169

S

self, 18–19, 36, 40–41, 74–75, 78, 83, 85–87, 101, 104–6, 108, 112, 145–46, 179, 183
self-dialogues, 54, 143
singing, 6, 10–11, 31, 57, 59, 131, 145
socialization, 39–41, 163
sounds, 16, 20–21, 23, 29, 44, 50, 55, 58–59, 61–63, 71, 90, 164, 168, 178, 180
space, 8, 13, 22, 30, 35, 50, 58, 61, 66, 69, 121, 130, 139, 159–60
spectacle, 94, 129, 131–32, 143, 147, 158
spectator, 124, 129, 159
stepping, 114–16, 132, 152, 158
stories, 50–52, 127, 129
strangeness, 82, 101–2, 111, 123, 132, 156
synchronization, 31, 33, 65–66, 147, 158–59

T

tensions, 46, 67, 102, 106, 122, 130, 132–33, 136–39, 142–43, 146–47, 157–58, 171
thinking, 4, 7, 38, 41–42, 58, 73–74, 91, 104, 149, 161, 164–65, 172–73
timing, 19, 23, 30–32, 140
truth, 84, 90, 92, 98, 108, 119, 130, 150, 157, 177

V

ventriloquism, 81, 90, 145, 150
voices, 50, 52–54, 57–59, 62, 64, 86–87, 89–90, 94, 118–19, 121–22, 145, 150, 152–53, 159, 182